Insights into Neurorehabilitation

Insights into Neurorehabilitation

By

Pengxu Wei

Cambridge
Scholars
Publishing

Insights into Neurorehabilitation

By Pengxu Wei

This book first published 2023

Cambridge Scholars Publishing

Lady Stephenson Library, Newcastle upon Tyne, NE6 2PA, UK

British Library Cataloguing in Publication Data
A catalogue record for this book is available from the British Library

ISBN (10): 1-5275-9084-4
ISBN (13): 978-1-5275-9084-7

TABLE OF CONTENTS

EMOTION-DRIVEN MOTIVATION IS CRUCIAL FOR MOTOR CONTROL

Key questions

- What is the neural substrate for emotion–motion interaction?
- What is the unique role of the cingulate motor area in motor control among cerebral motor cortices?

During motor rehabilitation, it is often found that patients are more willing to complete motor training tasks integrated into fun games in comparison with conventional training programs. Therefore, various games are increasingly applied in motor rehabilitation, including EMG biofeedback games and virtual reality games. The positive effects of emotional stimuli provided by the games indicate that emotion plays an important role in motor training and motor rehabilitation.

Origination of Brain motor cortices

Structure of the frontal lobe

The human frontal lobe consists of the prefrontal cortex, frontal eye fields, premotor cortices, and primary motor cortex (M1). The prefrontal cortex (PFC) is located on the most anterior portion of the frontal lobe medially, laterally, and orbitally. On the lateral side of the brain, the frontal lobe is located rostral to the central sulcus. In the frontal lobe, the lateral prefrontal cortex, frontal eye fields, premotor cortex, and primary motor cortex lie in a rostral to caudal order.

The dorsolateral prefrontal cortex (DLPFC) covers the entire dorsolateral surface of the frontal lobe, including most parts of the superior, middle, and inferior frontal gyri. The DLPFC is bounded posteriorly by several brain motor areas. The superior frontal gyrus consists of the prefrontal cortex, pre-supplementary motor cortex (pre-SMA), and supplementary motor cortex (SMA) from rostral to caudal.

The medial prefrontal cortex (mPFC) lies on the entire medial surface of the frontal lobe and envelops the corpus callosum ventrally, anteriorly, and dorsally (and thus the anterior cingulate cortex, ACC, is included) [1]. However, in some literature, on the medial side of the brain, the paracingulate sulcus is considered as (roughly) the border between the frontal lobe and the cingulate cortex of the limbic lobe (and thus ACC is not included) [2]. The cingulate motor cortex lies in the dorsal/middle portion of the cingulate cortex. The primary motor cortex is called M1, the supplementary motor cortex called M2, the rostral cingulate motor cortex called M3, and the caudal cingulate motor cortex called M4, though M2, M3, and M4 are rarely seen in recent literature.

The ventral part of the frontal lobe is the orbitofrontal cortex (OFC), which is located on the floor of the anterior cranial fossa, just above the orbits [2]. Orbital-ventromedial Prefrontal Cortex Contributes to Emotional Control of Behavior [1, 3.

Projections of brain areas in the frontal lobe

Orbitofrontal cortex (OFC)

The OFC receives inputs from all five types of sensory modalities and from the viscera.

1) The primary olfactory and gustatory cortices (mainly the insula) send olfactory and gustatory projections to the posterior OFC.
2) Unimodal parietal/temporal association areas (responsible for each sensory modality) send visual/somatosensory/auditory signals to the OFC. Especially, the somatosensory cortex sends somatosensory inputs in terms of mouth and hands, possibly indicating a role in feeding.
3) The nucleus of the solitary tract sends the fullness sensation to the OFC through the ventroposterior medial thalamus and agranular insula.

These inputs reach the posterior OFC and then are relayed to anterior OFC regions.

All three pathways relay appetitive- and feeding-related inputs (smell and taste of food, somatosensory information of mouth and hands, and fullness). In humans, feeding-related information and other rewarding stimuli are represented in the OFC [4].

Medial prefrontal cortex (mPFC)

The ventral mPFC areas receive inputs from the OFC. The dorsal mPFC areas receive inputs from the DLPFC. The ACC receives inputs from other mPFC areas and from the posterior cingulate cortex and parietal and temporal association cortices. Additionally, the mPFC receives relatively strong dopaminergic and serotonergic projections. The output projections of the mPFC reach the thalamus, amygdala, entorhinal cortex, and subiculum. Additionally, there is a unique relationship between the mPFC and subcortical brain areas related to the autonomic nervous system including the hypothalamus, PAG, and the dopaminergic, serotonergic, and noradrenergic brainstem nuclei.

These connections indicate that the mPFC is involved in the emotional processing of sensory stimuli. Abnormalities of the mPFC are detected in mood disorders, schizophrenia, substance use, and some other psychiatric problems [1].

Dorsolateral prefrontal cortex (DLPFC)

The DLPFC receives projection from multimodal association cortices, including the parietal lobe (somatosensory and visuospatial ["where" visual stream] information), and temporal lobe (auditory and visual object related information ["what" visual stream]. Strong dopaminergic and serotonergic inputs also reach the DLPFC.

DLPFC outputs mainly arrive at adjacent brain motor areas, that is, the M1, PMd, PMv, and SMA. It also connects the thalamus, striatum, and medial temporal lobe (MTL). The MTL encodes/ stores/retrieves specific memories, and marks the emotional values of the object and situation (the OFC and mPFC have stronger projections to the MTL than the DLPFC).

Such connections indicate that the DLPFC is closely related to cognitive processing rather than emotional and autonomic functions.

Function of motor cortices

- The prefrontal cortex (PFC) maintains the intention of goal-directed movements. Patients with a lesion in the PFC cannot remember their intentions and thus may devise plans one by one but abandon them immediately [3].
- Premotor cortices form motor plans, that is, generating an "abstract representation" of an intended motor action, e.g., which combination of limbs will be used or what is the sequence of movements.
- SMA and pre-SMA play a key role in selecting appropriate actions based on internal and external contexts. Lesions in this region lead to difficulties in initiating/suppressing movement. The initiation deficits manifest the loss of self-initiated movements of contralesional limbs or speech; the suppression deficits manifest the release phenomena, e.g., forced grasping when the hand touches an item, irrepressible reaching/searching movements towards an object), and the hand of the patient moving without being directed by the patient's own will.
- M1 execute skilled motor acts.

To sum up, in the frontal lobe, all brain areas participate in the motor control process. These areas are connected in series, forming a functional hierarchy. The dorsolateral prefrontal cortex (DLPFC) is responsible for the cognitive control of movement, especially the intention to perform movements. The signal then flows from the DLPFC to the premotor cortex (PMd, PMv, and SMC) and finally reaches M1 [3].

Emotion and cingulate cortex

The cingulate cortex is a neural interface between emotion, motivation, reward, sensation, and action, which is achieved by anatomical connections between the cingulate cortex and brain regions closely associated with each of such functions [5-8].

The exact functional subregions of the cingulate cortex remain unclear. Base on cytoarchitecture features, Brodman's area 24 is often referred to as anterior cingulate cortex (ACC) whereas Brodman's areas 23 and 31 are referred to as posterior cingulate cortex (PCC) [5, 9, 10]. As an alternative, the cingulate cortex may be divided into the ACC, MCC (middle cingulate cortex), and PCC [11]. Therefore, some parts of the MCC may be introduced as the ACC in other studies [12].

Motor tasks often evoke activations in the middle part of the cingulate cortex, a region called the cingulate motor area (CMA). The CMA is located mainly in the scope of the MCC whereas more anterior and posterior extensions may appear in movement-evoked activations [13, 14].

Several motor cortices participate in motor control. Through direct corticospinal projections, the primary motor cortex (M1) controls fractionated movements to execute a skilled motor act, such as opposing fingers to pick up a pen [14]. Projecting directly to the spinal cord, the dorsal and ventral premotor cortices (PMd and PMv, respectively), supplementary motor area (SMA, or more broadly, SMA and preSMA, called supplementary motor complex, SMC), and cingulate motor area (CMA) are main premotor areas that encode a general goal-directed command of a motor action. A motor task is thought to be divided into multiple subtasks, with each subtask managed in parallel by one of the cortical motor areas [15]. Then, a project is formed to move the fingers in the premotor areas. PMd has roles in movement preparation and guidance where PMV appears to play a major role in visually guided arm movements. SMA is responsible for initiating, programming, and planning movements [16]. M1 executes the movement. However, the role of CMA in brain motor control largely remains unclear. Neural activities in SMA and CMA are reported to be very similar during movement [17]. As a cortical region near SMA and sharing similar neural activities with SMA in motor control, the question of whether CMA has any unique function compared with those of SMA and other premotor areas should be answered.

Here, we directly compare the activation scopes evoked by stimulation/tasks rather than tangle with the nomenclature (ACC and PCC vs. ACC, MCC, and PCC). The emotion/motivation-evoked activity in the cingulate cortex is found to overlap those evoked by motor tasks: emotion/motivation-evoked activity are distributed over the anterior, middle, and posterior parts of the cingulate cortex, whereas activities evoked by motor tasks are distributed mainly in middle and anterior parts of the cingulate cortex (called cingulate motor area, CMA) [11, 12]. For example, motivation-induced brain activities are detected in the anterior and middle parts of the cingulate cortex [18], whereas the middle part can also be activated by motor tasks [13, 14].

The functional overlap suggests that the CMA may bridge the brain emotional/motivation processing network and motor control network. This is supported by several lines of evidence. First, stimulating the MCC/CMA region evokes both affective and motor responses [19].

Furthermore, brain activations in the MCC/CMA are observed in emotional (gentle or rude) hand movements, by using the direct contrast of gentle (or rude) hand movements vs. controlled hand movements. That is, MCC/CMA activations found in the study contain two parts, those evoked by the motor component of the hand movements and those evoked by the emotional component [20]. Additionally, emotion stimuli were found to evoke signal changes in the amygdala, middle insula, and MCC in a functional MRI study, whereas only the MCC activity presented a pattern similar to observed motor behavior changes, indicating that among all three emotion brain regions, only the MCC is closely related to motor outputs [21]. All these findings are direct evidence that MCC/CMA is a hub to integrate emotional and motor processing. In the brain motor areas, this role is unique.

The convergence of brain emotional network and motor network in MCC/CMA can be achieved by connections among MCC/CMA and other brain regions. A subregion of the cingulate cortex presents most strongly anatomical/functional connects to its adjacent brain areas and therefore possesses similar functions. For example, the posterior ACC is located adjacent to the orbitofrontal cortex, and both are responsible for emotional and motivational information processing. The dorsal ACC is adjacent to the lateral prefrontal cortex and pre-SMA, and all of them are involved in abstract cognitive processes. The MCC, overlapping the scope of the CMA, is adjacent to the SMA and M1, all of which participate in motor control. The posterior cingulate and retrosplenial cortex are located adjacent to the parietal and parahippocampal regions, and both process spatial information [5].

Each portion of the cingulate cortex also connects other brain regions in addition to those immediately adjacent areas. The cingulate cortex performs emotional and motivational processing via strong reciprocal projections to brain areas related to reward processing, e.g., the orbitofrontal cortex, basal ganglia, insula, and lateral prefrontal cortex [5]. Strong reciprocal connections also exist between the cingulate cortex and brain motor areas. Specifically, the MCC not only projects to M1, SMA, putamen, and spinal cord [22], but receives direct/indirect inputs from emotion-processing brain areas [23]. Connectivity analysis demonstrates that the MCC links the prefrontal and premotor cortices in addition to the M1 and SMA [19].

Therefore, the connections between the cingulate cortex and emotion/motivation/reward-processing brain areas and connections between the cingulate cortex and brain motor areas, especially the MCC, endow the CMA as a hub to bridge brain motor and emotion-motivation networks. Such a role well explains the unique function of the CMA in the brain motor system.

Emotion influences motor behavior to meet various needs, from basic survival requirements to social activities. Emotion concepts are critical in choosing appropriate actions and maintaining ongoing physiological balance [24]. Basic survival needs, such as food intake and predatory hunting, are regulated by the amygdala, which performs a primary role in processing emotional responses [25, 26]. Adolescents with a stronger emotion-driven impulsiveness tendency show a higher snacking frequency [27]. Unpleasant stimuli generate better force output in both healthy people and patients suffering from functional neurological symptom disorders than do pleasant stimuli [28]. In sports science, pleasant emotions such as happiness are thought to be associated with poor performance, whereas unpleasant emotions such as anxiety and anger are associated with good performance [29]. Emotion can even guide actions in ways we are often unaware of. For instance, although the task of dog owners walking their dog appears to be constructed as "for the dog", dog owners represent the dog's needs in a hidden manner, which is actually aligned with their own. The most important reason for dog walking is to meet the emotional needs of the owner rather than as a requirement for the dog's physical activity [30].

Movement also influences emotion. Walking or ergometer cycling positively affects depression and anxiety [31, 32]. High-intensity exercise leads to greater enjoyment due to elevated feelings of reward, excitement, and success than moderate-intensity exercise [33]. This result indicates a dose-dependent effect of movement on emotion. By contrast, inactivity due to bed rest for 10 days induces a decrease in positive emotions in healthy people [34].

Human behavior is either heavily influenced or motivated by emotions [35, 36]. Movement is a process in which motivation is actualized. PMd, PMv, and SMA are brain regions that plan and prepare motor acts, while M1 executes movements. CMA acts as a key area that introduces emotion–motivation drives to the brain motor system. Thus, the role of CMA is different from those of SMA, PMd, and PMv.

Brain emotion network may exert motivation to drive the brain motor network via CMA during non-emotional situations. This driving effect is supported by a previous finding that the directional ACC→SMA influence is greater during the motor task state than in the resting state in non-emotional situations [37]. The driving effect of emotion on motor outputs is also supported by the fact that amygdala neurons generate motivation for movement during situations without emotional stimuli [25].

To sum up, brain emotion and motor systems are tightly integrated; they are not only hard-wired in the brain across jawed vertebrates [25] but are seen among brain regions as revealed with functional MRI [38] and in the behavioral level [28, 30, 33, 34, 39]. CMA (mainly in MCC) bridges brain motor and emotion networks, thereby providing a neural substrate for emotion–motion interaction. With the CMA, the emotion network drives the brain motor system. Such a driving role may be explicit or latent, depending on the nature and magnitude of emotional changes. Thus, CMA plays a different role in motor control compared with other promotor areas such as SMA.

Emotion is the basic component of brain motor outputs

The brain emotion system influences the motor system in many ways. In the frontal lobe, the initiation to exert a motor behavior begins in the orbitofrontal-ventromedial prefrontal cortex (OFC and mPFC), and then flows along projections from the OFC and mPFC to the dorsolateral prefrontal cortex (DLPFC) [3]. Afterwards, the DLPFC mainly projects to the nearby motor, premotor, and supplementary motor areas. This OFC/mPFC-DLPFC-Premotor/SMC/M1 pathway represents an emotion-cognition-movement sequence in that the OFC/mPFC is more closely associated with emotional processing whereas the DLPFC is more closely associated with cognitive functions [1, 3]. This emotion-cognition-movement sequence also demonstrates the crucial role of emotion in initiating and controlling motor behavior. However, the CMA, as the interface/hub between brain emotional and motor systems, appears to directly integrate emotion and motor processing. The multi-level/area integration between brain emotional and motor systems strengthens the role of emotion, as a basic component, in brain motor control processing.

Emotion and motivation are closely related processes

Tomkins argued that emotion drives the behavior of a person as the basis of human motivation (to be concise, affect, emotion, and mood are not distinguished in this chapter). Motivation derived from the emotional system can amplify biological activities [40]. As an example, negative emotions including anxiety and depression can increase people's motivation to drink to achieve psychological relief [41, 42]. The concept that emotional systems act as the basic motivational system is supported by others [43]. Motivation and emotion systems in the brain share a number of common brain areas (e.g., the ACC and medial prefrontal cortex) and are tightly integrated [7, 18, 44], thereby often introduced together, e.g., the emotional-motivational system [45], emotional and motivational systems [43], emotional/motivational impact [46], and emotional-motivational brain functions [45].

The role of emotion/motivation in motor rehabilitation

Under most conditions, patients receive motor training via a cognitive process. That is, the medical professionals, caregivers, and patients realize the functional deficits and the necessities to restore the deficits. Then, a motor training course is given although the course may (and actually often) be boring, tedious, and lacking in variations. The course usually is composed of a number of motor tasks.

Because motor function deficits caused by a neurological disease (e.g., stroke) often lead to a heavy burden, patients usually follow the arrangement of the therapeutic exercise despite of abovementioned issues. However, the negative emotional status may lead to clinical problems to various extents, from mood swings to post-stroke depression. These problems impede the recovery of motor function and should be avoided. Thus, positive emotion should be built in a motor rehabilitation program, and negative emotion is to be avoided. In this way, the brain emotional system exerts a positive impact via CMA (and other brain emotion-motion interfaces) on the brain motor system, thereby promoting motivation to stick to motor training.

Practically, such a positive emotion-motivation impact can be achieved by using various approaches.

First, attractive content and appearance of the motor training program should be applied, such as adopting music, dance, and action video games in motor training. Music can lead to mood improvement [45], which improves emotional/motivational status and motor function in stroke patients [47]. The action video games are far more fun than the "boring" games commonly seen in healthcare facilities for training various functions of the patient. An example of an attractive appearance can be seen in a dolphin game (http://blam-lab.org/index.php/kata-design-studio/). The lifelike dolphin in the game exhibits a vivid, lively appearance, which can stimulate the interests of the patients. If possible, the motor training program should be designed and implemented as games instead of motor "tasks". A task implies a piece of work to be undertaken, whereas playing games is an activity for enjoyment rather than work and thus tends to cultivate initiative and even enthusiasm.

Secondly, challenge/difficulty levels of the contents of motor training should be carefully adopted. Similar to playing a game, a suitable challenge level can inspire participation whereas a level being too hard or too easy is hardly attractive for the patient. For example, when performing motor rehabilitation, the ability of a patient should be examined and the optimal level should be determined. Afterwards, the challenge/difficulty level of the motor action can be slightly increased beyond the optimal level, step by step. When successfully completing each training action one by one, the patient experience a series of success, and the motivation to keep training can be built. Such a process does not imply adopting challenges easy to be overcome. Instead, a challenge that can be overcome by using a certain amount of effort is preferred, which may induce a stronger imprint in the nervous system than easy-come-easy-go changes.

Additionally, the feedback should be timely presented to patients. A simple way to use feedback in motor training is to indicate muscle activities or limb movements with some type of biological signals, e.g., surface electromyography. However, an advanced approach is to determine the key components of a motor action, and trace its activity when performing motor training; the training may be to activate the muscle (from no voluntary muscle contractions to presenting stable voluntary contractions and from weak voluntary contractions to strong voluntary contractions) and to enhance functionality (improving endurance, selectivity, and dexterity of muscle contraction). Endurance is the ability to maintain enough duration when a muscle contracts; selectivity is the ability to contract relevant muscles but not irrelevant muscles for a motor action; dexterity indicates skillful rather than rigid or jerky movements and the ability to switch among concentric, eccentric, and isometric contractions. In each training session, no matter how tiny the progress is, the progress should be timely presented to the patients. The functional improvement can invigorate the patient if the function of the patient is continuously improved and positive feedback is timely given. As previously introduced, tight interaction exists among brain emotion and motivation systems. Additionally, the central role of the cingulate cortex in emotional- motivational processing is highlighted by its strong reciprocal connections to brain reward centers including the orbitofrontal cortex, basal ganglia, and insula, e.g., the ACC is the main target area of midbrain dopamine neurons and these neurons release dopamine to modulate reward responses [5]. Thus, the positive emotional/motivational modulation stemmed from a properly arranged training program and feedback can activate reward mechanisms, which enhances the impact of the emotion-motivation systems on brain motor outputs.

Summary

Human movements can be cognitively and/or emotionally motivated. It is a cognitive process to learn the possible effects of motor training on motor function recovery after neurological diseases such as stroke, which drive the compliance of a patient to receive training. Emotion-driven motivation may be explicit or latent and has a crucial impact on motor output because the brain emotion network and motor control network are tightly integrated via the CMA and other interfaces/hubs where the two systems converge. Thus, in motor training programs, positive emotions should be built to optimize the effect of therapeutic exercise.

References

[1] Stern TA, Rosenbaum JF, Fava M, Biederman J, Rauch SL. Massachusetts General Hospital Comprehensive Clinical Psychiatry. 2008. Philadelphia, USA. Mosby. 975-1124.

[2] Ramachandran VS. Encyclopedia of the Human Brain. 2002. 1st. San Diego. Academic Press. 11-14.

[3] Rizzolatti G, Kalaska JF. Principles of Neural Science. In: Kandel ER, Schwartz JH, Jessell TM, Siegelbaum SA, Hudspeth AJ eds. Principles of Neural Science. 2013. London. McGraw-Hill. 405-456.

[4] OngOngatti G, Kalaska JF. Principles of Neural Science. In: Kandel ER, Schwartz JH, Jessell rtex of rats, monkeys and humans. Cereb Cortex. 2000; 10: 206-19.

[5] Squire LR. Encyclopedia of Neuroscience. 2009. 1st. San Diego, USA. Elsevier Ltd. 887-892.

[6] Apps MA, Rushworth MF, Chang SW. The Anterior Cingulate Gyrus and Social Cognition: Tracking the Motivation of Others. Neuron. 2016； 90: 692-707.

[7] O'Reilly RC. Unraveling the Mysteries of Motivation. Trends Cogn Sci. 2020； 24: 425-434.

[8] Deng Y, Li S, Zhou R, Walter M. Motivation but not valence modulates neuroticism-dependent cingulate cortex and insula activity. Hum Brain Mapp. 2018； 39: 1664-1672.

[9] Johansen-Berg H, Behrens TEJ. Diffusion MRI From Quantitative Measurement to In vivo Neuroanatomy. 2014. 2nd. London, UK. Elsevier Inc. 481-509.

[10] Leech R, Sharp DJ. The role of the posterior cingulate cortex in cognition and disease. Brain. 2014 ； 137: 12-32. doi: 10.1093/brain/awt162.

[11] Vogt BA, Berger GR, Derbyshire SW. Structural and functional dichotomy of human midcingulate cortex. Eur J Neurosci. 2003； 18: 3134-44.

[12] Etkin A, Egner T, Kalisch R. Emotional processing in anterior cingulate and medial prefrontal cortex. Trends Cogn Sci. 2011； 15: 85-93 - 10.1016/j.tics.2010.11.004 [doi].

[13] Wei P, Zhang Z, Lv Z, Jing B. Strong Functional Connectivity among Homotopic Brain Areas Is Vital for Motor Control in Unilateral Limb Movement. Front Hum Neurosci. 2017； 11: 366 - 10.3389/fnhum.2017.00366 [doi].

[14] Wei P, Bao R, Lv Z, Jing B. Weak but Critical Links between Primary Somatosensory Centers and Motor Cortex during Movement. Front Hum Neurosci. 2018； 12: 1 - 10.3389/fnhum.2018.00001 [doi].

[15] Kandel E, Schwartz J, Jessell T. Principles of neural science. 2000. 4. Beijing. McGraw-Hill Medical. 674-712.

[16] Ramachandran VS. Encyclopedia of the Human Brain. 2002. 1st. San Diego. Academic Press. 11-14.

[17] Russo GS, Backus DA, Ye S, Crutcher MD. Neural activity in monkey dorsal and ventral cingulate motor areas: comparison with the supplementary motor area. J Neurophysiol. 2002; 88: 2612-29. doi: 10.1152/jn.00306.2002.

[18] Mattan BD, Kubota JT, Li T, Dang TP, Cloutier J. Motivation Modulates Brain Networks in Response to Faces Varying in Race and Status: A Multivariate Approach. eNeuro. 2018 ; 5. doi: 10.1523/ENEURO.0039-18.2018. eCollection 2018 Jul-Aug.

[19] Oane I, Barborica A, Chetan F, et al. Cingulate cortex function and multi-modal connectivity mapped using intracranial stimulation. Neuroimage. 2020; 220: 117059.

[20] Di Cesare G, Marchi M, Lombardi G, Gerbella M, Sciutti A, Rizzolatti G. The middle cingulate cortex and dorso-central insula: A mirror circuit encoding observation and execution of vitality forms. Proc Natl Acad Sci USA. 2021; 118. doi: 10.1073/pnas.2111358118.

[21] Pereira MG, de Oliveira L, Erthal FS, et al. Emotion affects action: Midcingulate cortex as a pivotal node of interaction between negative emotion and motor signals. Cogn Affect Behav Neurosci. 2010; 10: 94-106.

[22] Morecraft RJ, Louie JL, Schroeder CM, Avramov K. Segregated parallel inputs to the brachial spinal cord from the cingulate motor cortex in the monkey. Neuroreport. 1997; 8: 3933-8.

[23] Paus T. Primate anterior cingulate cortex: where motor control, drive and cognition interface. Nat Rev Neurosci. 2001; 2: 417-24. doi: 10.1038/35077500.

[24] Atzil S, Gendron M. Bio-behavioral synchrony promotes the development of conceptualized emotions. Curr Opin Psychol. 2017; 17: 162-169.

[25] Han W, Tellez LA, Rangel MJ Jr, et al. Integrated Control of Predatory Hunting by the Central Nucleus of the Amygdala. Cell. 2017; 168: 311-324.e18.

[26] Volkow ND, Wang GJ, Baler RD. Reward, dopamine and the control of food intake: implications for obesity. Trends Cogn Sci. 2011; 15: 37-46 - 10.1016/j.tics.2010.11.001 [doi].

[27] Coumans J, Danner UN, Intemann T, et al. Emotion-driven impulsiveness and snack food consumption of European adolescents: Results from the I.Family study. Appetite. 2018; 123: 152-159.

[28] Blakemore RL, Sinanaj I, Galli S, Aybek S, Vuilleumier P. Aversive stimuli exacerbate defensive motor behaviour in motor conversion disorder. Neuropsychologia. 2016; 93: 229-241 doi: 10.1016/j.neuropsychologia.2016.11.005..

[29] Lane AM, Beedie CJ, Jones MV, Uphill M, Devonport TJ. The BASES expert statement on emotion regulation in sport. J Sports Sci. 2012; 30: 1189-95.

[30] Westgarth C, Christley RM, Marvin G, Perkins E. I Walk My Dog Because It Makes Me Happy: A Qualitative Study to Understand Why Dogs Motivate Walking and Improved Health. Int J Environ Res Public Health. 2017; 14. - 10.3390/ijerph14080936 [doi].

[31] Vancini RL, Rayes A, Lira C, Sarro KJ, Andrade MS. Pilates and aerobic training improve levels of depression, anxiety and quality of life in overweight and obese individuals. Arq Neuropsiquiatr. 2017; 75: 850-857 doi: 10.1590/0004-282X20170149..

[32] Verschueren S, Eskes AM, Maaskant JM, Roest AM, Latour C, Op Reimer WS. The effect of exercise therapy on depressive and anxious symptoms in patients with ischemic heart disease: A systematic review. J Psychosom Res. 2018; 105: 80-91 doi: 10.1016/j.jpsychores.2017.11.018.

[33] Malik AA, Williams CAAOho, Bond B, Weston KL, Barker ARAOho. Acute cardiorespiratory, perceptual and enjoyment responses to high-intensity interval exercise in adolescents. Eur J Sport Sci. 2017; 17: 1335-1342 - 10.1080/17461391.2017.1364300 [doi].

[34] Stavrou NA, McDonnell AC, Eiken O, Mekjavic IB. Psychological strain: examining the effect of hypoxic bedrest and confinement. Physiol Behav. 2015; 139: 497-504 10.1016/j.physbeh.2014.12.015 [doi].

[35] Adolphs R. The social brain: neural basis of social knowledge. Annu Rev Psychol. 2009; 60: 693-716 – 10.1146/annurev.psych.60.110707.1635.

[36] Tomkins S. Affect Imagery Consciousness. 1962. 1st. New York. Springer. 28-118.

[37] Diwadkar VA, Asemi A, Burgess A, Chowdury A, Bressler SL. Potentiation of motor sub-networks for motor control but not working memory: Interaction of dACC and SMA revealed by resting-state directed functional connectivity. PLoS One. 2017; 12:

e0172531.

[38] Dreyer FR, Pulvermuller F. Abstract semantics in the motor system? - An event-related fMRI study on passive reading of semantic word categories carrying abstract emotional and mental meaning. Cortex. 2018; 100: 52-70 doi: 10.1016/j.cortex.2017.10.021.

[39] Coumans J, Danner UN, Intemann T, et al. Emotion-driven impulsiveness and snack food consumption of European adolescents: Results from the I.Family study. Appetite. 2018; 123: 152-159. doi: 10.1016/j.appet.2017.12.018.

[40] Holinger PC. Winnicott, Tomkins, and the Psychology of Affect. Clinical Social Work Journal. 2009; 37: 155.

[41] Peirce RS, Frone MR, Russell M, Cooper ML. Relationship of financial strain and psychosocial resources to alcohol use and abuse: the mediating role of negative affect and drinking motives. J Health Soc Behav. 1994; 35: 291-308.

[42] Pearlin LI, Radabaugh CW. Economic strains and the coping functions of alcohol. AJS. 1976; 82: 652-663. doi: 10.1086/226357.

[43] Żechowski C. Theory of drives and emotions - from Sigmund Freud to Jaak Panksepp. Psychiatr Pol. 2017 ; 51: 1181-1189. doi: 10.12740/PP/61781.

[44] Xu P, Chen A, Li Y, Xing X, Lu H. Medial prefrontal cortex in neurological diseases. Physiol Genomics. 2019; 51: 432-442. doi: 10.1152/physiolgenomics.00006.2019.

[45] Groenewegen HJ. The basal ganglia and motor control. Neural Plast. 2003; 10: 107-20. doi: 10.1155/NP.2003.107.

[46] Cogan ES, Shapses MA, Robinson TE, Tronson NC. Disrupting reconsolidation: memory erasure or blunting of emotional/motivational

value. Neuropsychopharmacology. 2019； 44: 399-407. doi: 10.1038/s41386-018-0082-0.

[47] Raglio A, Zaliani A, Baiardi P, et al. Active music therapy approach for stroke patients in the post-acute rehabilitation. Neurol Sci. 2017； 38: 893-897.

ARE HUMAN WALKING CPG IMPORTANT FOR WALKING TRAINING?

Key questions

- What is the neural mechanism of human walking?
- How to restore walking function after stroke or other neurological diseases leading to limb paralysis?
- Is the spinal CPG a target for training walking?
- Are body weight support treadmills and walking robotics useful for human walking training?

Spinal CPG alone cannot drive normal walking in adults

Rhythmic movement is a basic type of movement in humans and many animals, such as walking, running, breathing, chewing, swimming, and flapping wings during flight. Once initiated, rhythmic movements can be automatically repeated without intentional control to maintain the rhythm. The rhythmic activity originates from rhythmic action potentials generated by neurons in the central pattern generator (CPG). The CPG neurons may burst rhythmically spontaneously or when neuromodulators (or neuromodulatory substances) present [1-3]. In the circuits of a CPG, a small number of neurons generate strong rhythmic signals, whereas some neurons produce platform-shaped action potentials to exert effects over a relatively longer period [4].

Walking is one of the fundamental motor skills in humans. Rhythmic muscle activities, left–right alternating leg movements, and multi-joint movements of the lower limbs are core factors of human walking, which are considered the basic components of locomotion/walking movement patterns controlled by the CPG [5]. In animal experiments, these components are used to determine whether the lower limb motor actions are walking-like movements (and thus driven by the walking CPG). However, different from quadrupedal animals, a person must support the body and maintain balance during walking with two legs.

Previously, the alternating contractions of flexors and extensors of lower extremities during walking were considered as results of rhythmic activities in the central nervous circuits by which antagonistic muscle groups are suppressed by each other [6]. However, after removing timed sensory inputs, the locusts are still able to develop rhythmic movements (wing cycling) [7], suggesting that the rhythmic movement is not driven by spinal cord reflexes. In vertebrates such as Petromyzon [8] and neonatal rats [9], isolated spinal cords (or brainstem-spinal cord) can produce locomotion-like movements without peripheral sensory inputs, that is, periodically alternating left- and right-side contractions of the torso muscles (for Petromyzon) or extensor- and flexor-contractions of limb muscles (for rats).

The locomotion/walking CPG exists in the spinal cord in quadrupedal animals such as cats or rats. Walking-like movement patterns can spontaneously occur in decerebrated mammals [10], and the walking CPG in mammals comprises rhythm-generating and pattern-generating circuits in the spinal cord [11]. The rhythm-generating circuit consists of excitatory, ipsilaterally projecting interneurons to motivate the CPG and establish the pace of gait rhythms [12]. The pattern-generating circuit sends rhythmic drives to motor neuron pools in the spinal cord, generating a flexor-extensor alternating pattern and a left-right alternating pattern. The flexor-extensor alternating pattern coordinates intra-limb movements via ipsilaterally projecting interneurons, whereas the left-right alternating pattern controls inter-limb coordinated activities via commissural interneurons [11, 13, 14]. Notably, the leg flexors or extensors can be activated separately by rhythmic activities driven by spinal excitatory neurons alone [12], rather than by the reciprocal inhibition between antagonistic flexor- and extensor-related excitatory mechanisms [6].

The firing pattern of electromyographic (EMG) signals supports the existence of the spinal CPG to generate walking-like movement patterns in animals [8, 15]. However, such findings are detected in decerebrated/spinalized animals instead of intact mammals. For walking behavior in intact animals, the influence of supraspinal centers (i.e., brainstem and brain) and peripheral afferents cannot be excluded, and thus purely spinal CPG-controlled walking is unable to be acquired.

In a study recruiting motor-complete spinal cord injury patients, after single-dose administration of buspirone/levodopa/carbidopa (but not levodopa/carbidopa, buspirone, or placebo), walking-like movement patterns, that is, rhythmic flexor-extensor and left-right alternating muscle activities in lower limbs, can be detected [16]. This finding supports the existence of the walking CPGs in the human spinal cord.

In a gait cycle of neonates, EMG signals of lower limb and trunk muscles during assisted walking-like movements (continues, forward stepping) present two basic patterns. One pattern is extensor muscles coactivated during the stance phase and the other pattern is flexor muscles coactivated during the swing phase. The two patterns alternately appear during walking [17]. The two basic patterns are very similar to the basic extensor and flexor patterns identified in motor-complete spinal cord injury patients [18] and thus may be driven by the spinal CPG since supraspinal impacts can be excluded. For toddlers, preschoolers, and adults, the two basic patterns still exist during walking whereas two new patterns are complemented [17]. That is, the spinal CPG exerts function during walking from newborns to adults to generate two basic patterns to activate leg muscles, whereas new patterns during development are needed to achieve normal walking in adults. The new patterns are acquired motor skills learned/modulated by using supraspinal centers, that is, neural circuits in the brain and brainstem in healthy people.

Brain networks that control human walking

The single photon emission computed tomography (SPECT), positron emissiontomography (PET), functional magnetic resonance imaging (fMRI), functional near-infrared spectroscopy (fNIRS), electroencephalogram (EEG), and magnetoencephalography (MEG) are tools to explore brain functions. Of these techniques, fMRI holds relatively high spatial and temporal resolutions. Additionally, fMRI is the only feasible tool to examine brainstem functions at present.

When examining brain and brainstem networks to control normal walking in humans, movement paradigms applied in determining spinal CPGs should be applied, that is, a rhythmic, bilaterally involved, flexor-extensor alternating leg movement to simulate basic components of human walking. Such a paradigm has been used in previous studies, many involving ankle movements in a supine position [19-24].

Ankle movements with different speeds can be applied to provide variations, that is, slow-, fast-, and usual-speed walking. Based on the needs of specific contexts during walking, healthy persons can change the speed (or frequency) of steps. Here, several motor tasks with the basic components of human walking but different frequencies were adopted to build corresponding relationships between the applied motor tasks and different types of walking in real life. The simulated walking movements were paced by audio cues. A set of independent component analysis (ICA) parameters, which has been proven to generate highly reliable results [25], was applied to uncover brain networks controlling the simulated walking movements. Four consistent walking-control brain networks across all walking tasks were detected (**Figure 1**), that is, the cerebellum network, rhythm-control network (consisting of the PAC, S2, IPC, and preSMA), walking speed-differentiating network (consisting of the lateral S1, SPL, and PMd), and basic actor network (consisting of the medial primary somotosensorimotor cortices, SMA, premotor cortex, and SPL) [26].

In **Figure 1,** cerebellum network: red; rhythm-control network (PAC-S2-IPC-preSMA): yellow; basic actor network (medial M1S1-SMA-PreM-SPL): blue; walking speed-differentiating network (S1-SPL-PMd): purple. The numbers indicate MNI coordinates in the *z*-axis [26].

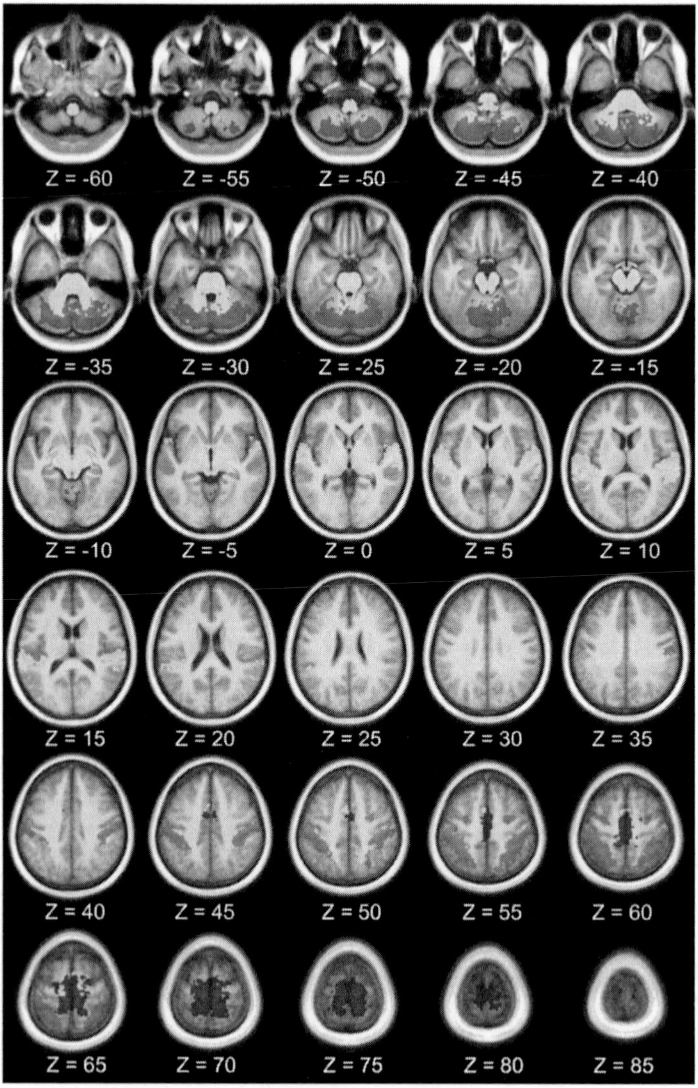

Figure 1. Four brain networks for walking control.

The rhythm-control network mainly covers the PAC, thereby presenting a primary role in dealing with audio information which sets the rhythm of the movements. All motor tasks in the study used audio cues to pace ankle movements. This network also covers some parts of the preSMA, a brain region proven to participate in chunking and related processes, such as task switching, response selection, and response inhibition when performing sequential movements [27]. For a sequential movement such as the (simulated) walking behavior, the preSMA separates the entire motor action into a number of minor fragments and is involved in switching such fragments. It appears that in this brain network, the preSMA exerts these functions by using audio cues processed in the PAC and sensory inputs from the S2 and IPC. The inferior temporal cortex preferentially participates in the cognitive aspects of discriminating shape and object, whereas the IPC plays roles in object-oriented action, object recognition, and motor planning [28]. Briefly, this network controls the rhythm of the simulated walking by integrating audio inputs (PAC), chunking/switching function (preSMA), and sensory processing in high-order sensory cortices (S2 and IPC).

The walking speed-differentiating network is distributed mainly in the parietal lobe, including the lateral parts of S1 and SPL, and covers a small part of PMd. This network exhibits a negative temporal correlation value with the time course of the ankle movements with slow speeds (0.5 and 1 Hz) but a positive temporal correlation value with the time course of higher-speed walking tasks (2 Hz, usual-speed, and changing-speed conditions), thereby indicating different roles in walking movements with a slow or high speed. According to the somatotopy revealed in a previous study [29], the lateral part of S1 in this network covers the representation area of body parts above the knees but not the lower leg. It appears that the lateral S1, SPL, and PMd in this network integrate somatosensory inputs from the body other than the moving part (in the lateral S1), movement preparation (in the PMd), and sensorimotor integration (in the SPL) to facilitate the involvement of the whole body during fast walking. During slowing walking, the network is deactivated.

The basic actor network is mainly distributed over the medial parts of M1 and covers the representation areas of the lower leg, including ankles and feet. These brain regions are commonly reported in previous fMRI studies on foot movements and are fundamental brain areas for motor execution and related sensory processing. Hence, this network exerts function as a basic actor to control walking movements. This basic actor network is found in all ankle movement conditions and in the resting state. The spatial map during the resting state covers more lateral parts of M1 and S1 than the map during task conditions. Such spatial inconsistency leads to low correlation values. The spatial map in the task conditions is only the medial part of the map in the resting state, possibly due to only the lower leg being involved in motor tasks [26].

The cerebellum network covers almost all parts of the cerebellum and exhibits the highest level of consistency across all motor tasks, thereby indicating a fundamental role in walking control. Compared with limb movements in simple ways such as a single unilateral ankle movement, the cerebellum is more likely to participate in modulating complicated movements such as bilaterally alternating ankle dorsiflexion/plantarflexion to simulate walking. Additionally, the cerebellum is also a place to modulate movements with somatosensory inputs [30, 31]. Complex motor actions such as walking need to process intensive somatosensory information for feedforward/feedback control. Therefore, this network covers extensive areas of the cerebellum.

These four networks exhibit a frame of how the adult human brain controls walking-like movements. Via these central mechanisms, the brain modulates lower centers in the brainstem and spinal cord to accommodate adjustments to meet internal and external needs during walking.

Walking-control mechanisms in the brainstem

Brainstem nuclei and circuits to control walking-like movements have also been detected (**Figure 2**) [32]. These findings confirm the role of the brainstem in human walking.

In the mesencephalic (or midbrain) locomotor region (MLR) of vertebrates, the pedunculopontine nucleus (PPN) is involved in controlling slow locomotion such as exploring nearby environments or searching for food, whereas the cuneiform nucleus (CN) controls faster speed locomotion such as running to escape from danger [33, 34]. Our findings support these roles of the CN and PPN in walking control in humans. Additionally, our results indicate that the simulated walking movements evoked brainstem activations in the red nucleus, and several pons and medulla areas besides the CN and PPN (**Figure 2**) [32], though the ventral pons was excluded due to susceptibility-induced blood-oxygen-level-dependent (BOLD) signals loss in this region in fMRI images [35].

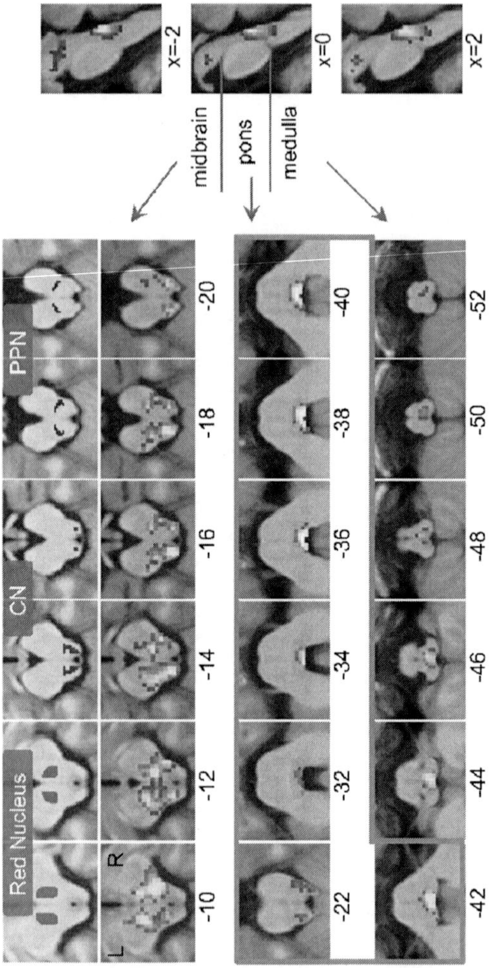

Figure 2. Brainstem structures during walking-like movements. Anatomical scopes of the CN, PPN, and red nucleus are presented in the first row. The images of the pons are framed in orange. Brainstem activation is projected onto the anatomical MRI image. The numbers on the x-axis (for the sagittal plane, on the right side) or the z-axis (for the axial plane, on the left side) indicate the MNI coordinate [32].

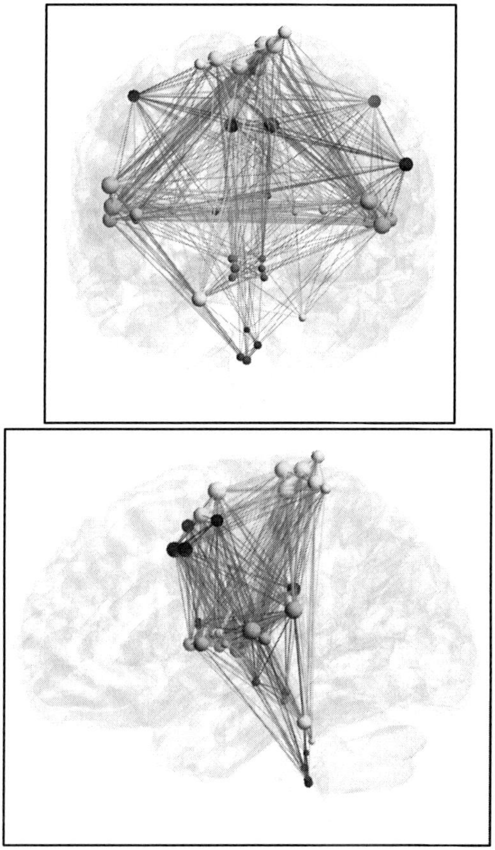

Figure 3. Two brainstem modules for human walking control. The brain/brainstem nodes in the same module are shown in the same color. Bilateral midbrain nodes (pink) and pons–medulla nodes (red) constitute two modules during usual-speed walking-like movements. Edges are sized according to their weight, and brain regions (nodes) are sized according to nodal strength (the sum of weights of all edges connected to this node). The smaller size of nodes and finer edges in a network indicate lower nodal strength and weaker internodal connections, respectively [32].

The activated brainstem regions can be classified into two modules (see [36] for the methodological background of ROI selection from activated brain regions). In a network, a module is a group of densely interconnected nodes (here are brain regions) that sparsely connect the remaining nodes in this network; a module can thus be regarded as a unit to exert a relatively independent function [37]. One detected module consists of bilateral CNs and PPNs where the other consists of the four pons–medulla regions. The two modules are found in all examined simulated-walking movements, thereby indicating two brainstem functional units existed across various walking conditions (**Figure 3** presents the two modules during simulated walking with a usual speed).

Walking Automaticity

Healthy adults walk in a way presenting high automaticity. For example, people often walk in a street while engaging in other activities, without attention to controlling walking movements [38]. Such automaticity is considered to rely on cortical control and lumbar spinal circuits (i.e., the spinal walking CPG) [5, 39].

It should be emphasized here that the four brain networks and the two brainstem circuits both commonly existed across all examined walking tasks. Thus, these networks/circuits are neural mechanisms to control the core components of walking rather than specific aspects of a given walking type. As previously introduced, the core components of human walking are the rhythmically alternating left-right, flexor-extensor, multi-joint movements of the lower limbs. It therefore can be concluded that the detected brain networks and brainstem circuits, together with the spinal CPG, form a generator in the entire central nervous system to drive the basic components of walking (i.e., rhythmically alternating left–right, flexor-extensor, and multi-joint movements of the lower limbs). No high-level cognitive centers (brain areas in the prefrontal cortex) exist in the four brain networks, even for the changing-speed condition requiring gait speed modulation, indicating that either simple walking (e.g., slow-, fast-, and usual-speed conditions) or more complex walking (e.g., changing-speed) tasks can be achieved without consuming constant high-level cognitive resources in the brain. That is also consistent with the concept that automaticity is a basic feature of walking in healthy humans.

However, such automaticity can be enhanced during the fast-speed and usual-speed walking tasks, e.g., the mismatch between a faster walking speed and a weaker brainstem–cortex interaction during fast-speed and usual-speed conditions supports a partially "automatic" gait control by the brainstem [32]. Such automaticity corresponds to stronger interactions among bilateral CNs, PPNs, and red nuclei (for fast-speed walking, bilateral thalami are also contained). The CN-PPN-red nucleus circuit, therefore, appears to be the neural substrate of walking automaticity at the level of the brainstem.

Generalized walking "CPG" in the central nervous system

When using rhythmically alternating left-right, flexor-extensor, multi-joint movements of the lower limbs as an activity to present core components of human walking, the existence of the spinal walking CPG is supported by behavioral and EMG findings in motor-complete spinal cord injury patients, who exhibit such walking-like movement patterns after administration of certain drugs [16]. In healthy young adults examined with fMRI, we find two brainstem circuits and four brain networks as the neural substrates of walking control. Taken together, the spinal walking CPG, two brainstem circuits, and four brain networks form a generalized walking "CPG" in the human central nervous system to maintain walking. The generalized walking "CPG" can accommodate some types of variations such as a constant slow or fast speed, or a changing walking speed; such central adaptability is partly represented by different brain and brainstem activating/organizing patterns across the varied walking status. For example, the spinal CPG alone can generate a wide range of rhythms ranging from 0.27–1.84 Hz [18]. To meet specific needs, the CN–PPN–red nucleus circuit participates in controlling a relative automatic gait control during faster locomotion in the brainstem, whereas the rhythm-control (PAC-S2-IPC-preSMA) network and walking speed-differentiating (S1-SPL-PMd) network modulate gait speed in the brain.

All these central neural control mechanisms are bilaterally involved. As previously introduced, the spinal CPG drives the flexor-extensor alternating pattern to coordinate intra-limb movements via ipsilaterally projecting interneurons and the left-right alternating pattern to control inter-limb coordination via commissural interneurons. In the midbrain, the CN–PPN–red nucleus circuit consists of bilaterally distributed structures. The four brain networks are also almost symmetrically distributed in bilateral cerebral and cerebellar hemispheres. Walking movements in healthy adults are also symmetrically performed movements by bilateral limbs. Nevertheless, hemiplegia patients cannot walk normally due to damaged brain control and secondary muscular dysfunction, and it is a challenge to reorganize the central nervous system to resume walking function.

Small modules in spinal CPG provide plasticity

In mice, the unilateral rhythmic locomotor activity of motor neurons in the spinal cord can be evoked. Furthermore, the leg flexors or extensors can be separately elicited by rhythmic activities driven by spinal excitatory neurons alone [12]. Thus, small modules to drive the rhythmic activity of leg flexors or extensors can be combined to generate alternating leg flexor-extensors activities. Broadly, the small modules can be recruited to produce unilateral and bilateral leg movements for walking. Such a modular distributed organization of the spinal CPG underlies flexibility or variability of walking-related neuromuscular activities to accommodate changes in walking during development or under different contexts. Hemiplegia patients may recruit some of these modules for walking independently. The pathological gaits may lose rhythm and present various abnormal patterns.

During walking, intentionally adjusting a biomechanical component of walking is hardly effective due to the automatic nature of walking behavior. In addition to the rhythmically alternating left-right, flexor-extensor, and multi-joint movements in the lower limbs, enough weight-bearing ability during the stance phase is another key element of human walking. In healthy adults, the weight-bearing and rhythmically alternating leg movements can be achieved during walking without intentional control.

When receiving motor training, an element of walking should be intervened separately and then integrated into ongoing walking training. For example, knee extensors may be strengthened to improve weight-bearing control during the stance phase by using stepping up/down stairs or position keeping when loading the body weight on one leg. It is not proper to focus on extending the knee during walking.

How weight-bearing is achieved during development

The two basic movement patterns derived from newborn babies (3.2 ± 1.4 days old) [17] are consistent with those decomposed from EMG data of motor-complete spinal cord injury patients (leftmost column of Figure 4 A in [18]). Both of them are two sinusoidal-like curves representing alternating leg extensor-flexor activities in a group of leg muscles, one as extensor coactivations and the other as flexor coactivations [17]. The two patterns shown in the provided video in [17] are consistent with synergistic movements of leg extensors/flexors (e.g., in stroke patients). Two new patterns, first appearing in toddlers (11-14 months old), then in preschoolers (22-48 months old), and finally in adults (25-40 years old), are one peaked at the early stance phase (foot strike/initial contact) in a gait cycle and the other peaked at early swing phase. Also note that during development, the shape of the sinusoidal-like extensor synergistic pattern is changed to a curve with a sharper peak at the midstance, and the shape of the sinusoidal-like flexor synergistic pattern is changed to a curve with a sharper peak at the end swing.

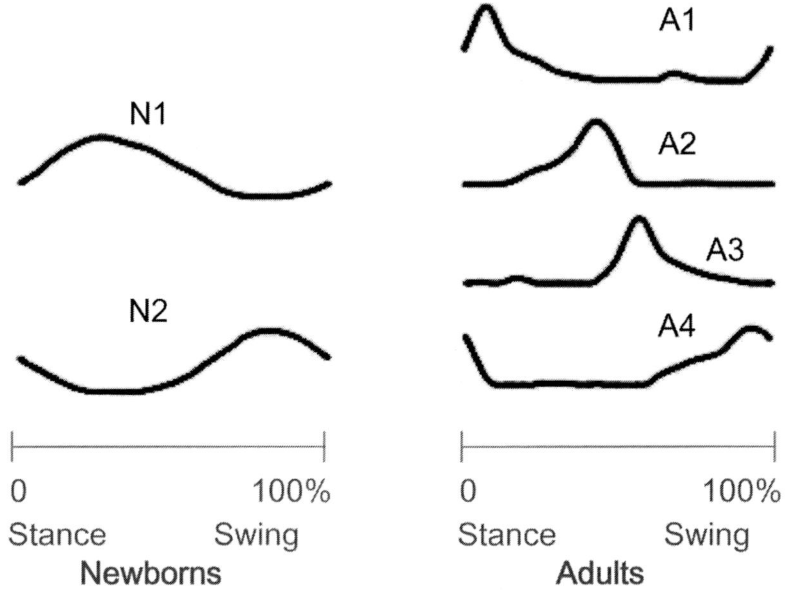

Figure 4. Activation patterns of neonates and adults in a gait cycle (right leg). N1: extensor coactivations of neonates; N2: flexor coactivations of neonates; A1: early-stance extensor activations of adults; A2: extensor coactivations of adults; A3: early swing flexor activations of adults; A4: flexor coactivations of adults. A1 is timed at initial contact/foot strike, A2 at weight acceptance, A3 at forward propulsion, and A4 at foot lift-off. The curves of the four patterns are drawn by referring to [17]).

The weight-bearing adaptation during development consists of two aspects, that is, from the extensor coactivations in neonates (N1) to an early-stance extensor activation (A1) and an extensor coactivation (A2) in adults. Similarly, the flexor coactivations in neonates (N2) are adapted to an early swing flexor activation (A3) and a flexor coactivation (A4) in adults to provide better flexion control during walking.

The difference between the two activation patterns in newborns and the four patterns in adults indicates that the spinal CPG alone can only drive two basic movement patterns but not the pattern for weight-bearing control. The weight-bearing pattern appearing during development are results of brain and brainstem modulation based on biomechanical requirements and sensory inputs during walking. Similarly, in motor-complete spinal cord injury patients, neither drug administration [16] nor spinal cord electrical stimulation [18] can elicit the weight-bearing capacity/pattern.

Due to the lack of weight-bearing adaptation, spinal CPG alone cannot achieve effective walking.

Weight-bearing is the key element for effective and safe walking and thus is of higher priority than rhythmic activities of lower limb muscles. The ability of weight bearing should be focused on as early as possible during motor rehabilitation. Effective weight-bearing capacity needs a series of special training.

In the aspects of neural control, the spinal cord consists of distributed modules to control activities of extensors/flexors, those rhythmically bursting leg extensors/flexors unilaterally, and those rhythmically coordinating bilateral leg movements. These spinal modules can be fine-tuned by brainstem and brain centers to achieve normal walking. The weight-bearing ability, though still lacking clear understood neural mechanisms, can be trained possibly via enhancing some spinal modules and modulation from brainstem and brain networks.

Methods to improve weight-bearing capacity

The weight-bearing ability, but not the rhythmically alternating flexor-extensor activities of bilateral legs, plays a primary role in human walking; otherwise, the standing body collapses. A hemiplegia patient can walk in a non-rhythmical manner even with little activities in leg flexors if the body can be well supported by the extensors and other muscles during locomotion. Thus, the primary goal when resuming walking function is to improve the weight-bearing ability of the patient. Without a strong enough weight-bearing function, the rhythmic leg muscle activities alone cannot achieve walking. Clinically, the weight-bearing can be trained by using a series of therapeutic exercises performed in upright positions.

After stroke, an example algorithm for restoring standing and walking ability is as follows: strengthening neck and trunk extensors via maintaining sitting positions in the early stage → bridge exercise in supine position to strengthen the trunk and hip extensors → standing exercise to strengthen whole-body extensors, particularly in lower limbs, → walking exercise with or without assistive devices, e.g., walkers or orthoses. If the alignment is well controlled, standing with body weight borne by the paralyzed leg is a very effective exercise to strengthen lower leg extensors. Notably, if a relative severe paralysis of the lower extremity exists, the benefit of a body-weight support system (treadmills or robotics) may not come from the rhythmic activity it provides but originate from the effects of dynamic weight-bearing. The hip extensors are often the first to exhibit function among leg extensors. Since the function of hip adductors is always recovered earlier than other hip movers, motor training may focus on hip extensors and then hip abductors (gluteus medius and gluteus minimus) for improving weight-bearing control and pelvic alignment in upright positions. Hip flexors can be exercised with special techniques if good weight-bearing is achieved and the patient has enough potential.

References

[1] Ryckebusch S, Laurent G. Rhythmic patterns evoked in locust leg motor neurons by the muscarinic agonist pilocarpine. J Neurophysiol. 1993; 69: 1583-95.

[2] Harris-Warrick RM, Flamm RE. Multiple mechanisms of bursting in a conditional bursting neuron. J Neurosci. 1987; 7: 2113-28.

[3] Hooper SL, Marder E. Modulation of the lobster pyloric rhythm by the peptide proctolin. J Neurosci. 1987; 7: 2097-112.

[4] Marder E, Bucher D. Central pattern generators and the control of rhythmic movements. Curr Biol. 2001; 11: R986-96.

[5] Minassian K, Hofstoetter US, Dzeladini F, Guertin PA, Ijspeert A. The Human Central Pattern Generator for Locomotion: Does It Exist and Contribute to Walking. Neuroscientist. 2017; 23: 649-663.

[6] Brown TG. On the nature of the fundamental activity of the nervous centres; together with an analysis of the conditioning of rhythmic activity in progression, and a theory of the evolution of function in the nervous system. J Physiol. 1914; 48: 18-46.

[7] WILSON DM. The Central Nervous Control of Flight in a Locust. Journal of Experimental Biology;J Exp Biol. 38(2) ,1961. 471 LP - 490.

[8] Grillner S. Neurobiological bases of rhythmic motor acts in vertebrates. Science. 1985; 228: 143-9.

[9] Cazalets JR, Sqalli-Houssaini Y, Clarac F. Activation of the central pattern generators for locomotion by serotonin and excitatory amino acids in neonatal rat. J Physiol. 1992; 455: 187-204.

[10] Frigon A. Central pattern generators of the mammalian spinal cord. Neuroscientist. 2012; 18: 56-69.

[11] Kiehn O. Decoding the organization of spinal circuits that control locomotion. Nat Rev Neurosci. 2016; 17: 224-38.

[12] Hägglund M, Dougherty KJ, Borgius L, Itohara S, Iwasato T, Kiehn O. Optogenetic dissection reveals multiple rhythmogenic modules underlying locomotion. Proc Natl Acad Sci USA. 2013; 110: 11589-94.

[13] Zhang J, Lanuza GM, Britz O, et al. V1 and v2b interneurons secure the alternating flexor-extensor motor activity mice require for limbed locomotion. Neuron. 2014; 82: 138-50.

[14] Talpalar AE, Endo T, Löw P, et al. Identification of minimal neuronal networks involved in flexor-extensor alternation in the mammalian spinal cord. Neuron. 2011; 71: 1071-84.

[15] Frigon A, Rossignol S. Experiments and models of sensorimotor interactions during locomotion. Biol Cybern. 2006; 95: 607-27.

[16] Radhakrishna M, Steuer I, Prince F, et al. Double-Blind, Placebo-Controlled, Randomized Phase I/IIa Study (Safety and Efficacy) with Buspirone/Levodopa/Carbidopa (SpinalonTM) in Subjects with Complete AIS A or Motor-Complete AIS B Spinal Cord Injury. Curr Pharm Des. 2017; 23: 1789-1804.

[17] Dominici N, Ivanenko YP, Cappellini G, et al. Locomotor primitives in newborn babies and their development. Science. 2011; 334: 997-9.

[18] Danner SM, Hofstoetter US, Freundl B, et al. Human spinal locomotor control is based on flexibly organized burst generators. Brain. 2015； 138: 577-88.

[19] CAUDA F. MR compatible device for active and passive foot movements. International Journal of Mechanics and Control. 11,2010

[20] Jaeger L, Marchal-Crespo L, Wolf P, Riener R, Michels L, Kollias S. Brain activation associated with active and passive lower limb stepping. Front Hum Neurosci. 2014. 8: 828.

[21] Newton JM, Dong Y, Hidler J, et al. Reliable assessment of lower limb motor representations with fMRI: use of a novel MR compatible device for real-time monitoring of ankle, knee and hip torques. Neuroimage. 2008. 43(1): 136-146.

[22] KAPRELI E, ATHANASOPOULOS S, PAPATHANASIOU M, et al. Lower limb sensorimotor network: issues of somatotopy and overlap[J]. Cortex; a journal devoted to the study of the nervous system and behavior, 2007, 43(2): 219-232

[23] Francis S, Lin X, Aboushoushah S, et al. fMRI analysis of active, passive and electrically stimulated ankle dorsiflexion. Neuroimage. 2009. 44(2): 469-479.

[24] Trinastic JP, Kautz SA, McGregor K, et al. An fMRI study of the differences in brain activity during active ankle dorsiflexion and plantarflexion. Brain Imaging Behav. 2010. 4(2): 121-131.

[25] Wei P, Bao R, Fan Y. Comparing the reliability of different ICA algorithms for fMRI analysis. PLoS One. 2022； 17: e0270556.

[26] Wei P, Zou T, Lv Z, Fan Y. Human locomotion-control brain networks detected with independent component analysis. J Integr

Neurosci. 2021； 20: 695-701.

[27] Xu B, Sandrini M, Wang WT, et al. PreSMA stimulation changes task-free functional connectivity in the fronto-basal-ganglia that correlates with response inhibition efficiency. Hum Brain Mapp. 2016； 37: 3236-49.

[28] Jancke L, Kleinschmidt A, Mirzazade S, Shah NJ, Freund HJ. The role of the inferior parietal cortex in linking the tactile perception and manual construction of object shapes. Cereb Cortex. 2001； 11: 114-21.

[29] Bao R, Wei P, Li K, et al. Within-limb somatotopic organization in human SI and parietal operculum for the leg: An fMRI study. Brain Res. 2012； .

[30] Ramachandran VS. Encyclopedia of the Human Brain, Volume 4. 2002. 1st. San Diego. Academic Press. 574-597.

[31] Standring S. Gray's Anatomy. 2004. 39. UK. Churchill Livingstone. 1104-1111.

[32] Wei P, Zou T, Lv Z, Fan Y. Functional MRI Reveals Locomotion-Control Neural Circuits in Human Brainstem. Brain Sci. 2020； 10.

[33] Ferreira-Pinto MJ, Ruder L, Capelli P, Arber S. Connecting Circuits for Supraspinal Control of Locomotion. Neuron. 2018； 100: 361-374.

[34] Caggiano V, Leiras R, Goni-Erro H, et al. Midbrain circuits that set locomotor speed and gait selection. Nature. 2018； 553: 455-460.

[35] Wei P, Lan Z, Lv Z, Fan Y. Brainstem fMRI. Encyclopedia. 2020； 1: 4-11.

[36] Wei P, Bao R, Fan Y. Independence of functional connectivity analysis in fMRI research does not rely on whether seeds are exogenous or endogenous. Medicine in Novel Technology and Devices. 2022； 15: 100126.

[37] Bassett DS, Wymbs NF, Porter MA, Mucha PJ, Carlson JM, Grafton ST. Dynamic reconfiguration of human brain networks during learning. Proc Natl Acad Sci USA. 2011； 108: 7641-6.

[38] Harms IM, van Dijken JH, Brookhuis KA, de Waard D. Walking Without Awareness. Front Psychol. 2019； 10: 1846.

[39] Sacheli LMAOho, Zapparoli L, Bonandrini R, et al. How aging affects the premotor control of lower limb movements in simulated gait. Hum Brain Mapp. 2020； 41: 1889-1903.

MOTOR TRAINING AFTER STROKE: AN APPROACH ORIENTED BY FORCE-EXERTING MODE

Key questions

- Are movement patterns and biomechanical components enough to describe the essence of human motor skills?
- Why is the force-exerting mode a "deeper" concept than movement patterns and biomechanical components?
- What are the key motor skills during motor training for hemiplegia due to upper motor neuron lesions such as stroke?

History of motor rehabilitation training after stroke

In adults, stroke (or cerebrovascular disease) ranks first in frequency and importance among all types of neurologic diseases. Stroke is a sudden focal neurologic syndrome caused by abnormalities of the brain resulting from a pathologic process of blood vessels, that is, the interruption of the blood supply to the brain because of a burst or blockage of the blood vessel. This blocks the supply of oxygen and nutrients, leading to brain tissue damage. The severity of a stroke depends on where the brain is injured and how severely it is damaged [1].

Stroke results in heavy burdens on the individual, family, and community. It is a leading cause of adult disability. Motor deficits are common after stroke. It is crucial to recover motor function for stroke patients to regain independence. However, recovery of motor function after stroke is always a challenge [2, 3].

Historically, there were transitions among representative concepts and techniques for stroke rehabilitation. From 1916 to 1955, the poliovirus infected an average of about 38 000 people each year in the United States. Such a huge amount of patients advanced the development of physical therapy and rehabilitation medicine. Treatments of this disease focused on the loss of flexibility, loss of muscle power, the potential for deformity, loss of skill, and other issues. Obviously, these approaches mainly focus on individual muscles (that is, muscle reeducation), since the poliovirus affects motor neurons of the brainstem and spinal cord, and produces the classic lower-motor neuron symptoms of paralysis, atrophy, and subsequent contracture [4, 5].

However, stroke leads to brain damage. The motor impairment after stroke has totally different manifestations in comparison with poliomyelitis. Based on the understanding of neurophysiology, neuroanatomy, and pathophysiology of stroke, several types of therapeutic exercise techniques were developed in approximately the 1950's, including the work of Bobaths, Brunnstrom, Rood, Kabat, Knott, and Voss. The concepts underlying these techniques were called the facilitation model. For decades, facilitation techniques were the mainstream in the motor rehabilitation program for stroke patients. After that, the clinical effect and theoretical basis of facilitation techniques were challenged. [5] New concepts and approaches have been developing, including biomechanical analysis and task-oriented concepts (represented by the motor relearning program), body weight support treadmill, mirror therapy, motor imagery, constraint-induced movement therapy, and robotics-assisted training. However, the therapeutic effects of current approaches are still not satisfactory.

For developing approaches to recover motor impairments in stroke patients, it is important to understand the nature of normal and impaired motor control and establish principles for designing methods to improve motor function. Here, several crucial issues are discussed.

Essence of developing motor skills

Motor skills of normal infants are developing. Newborn infants cannot sit, stand, and walk. In two months, they can lift heads almost 45 degrees when on stomachs. In four months, they can raise heads 90 degrees when placed on stomachs, and hold and release an object. In six months, infants are able to pick up a dropped object. In 12 months, they can pick up a small object using the tip of their thumb and index finger. A two-year-old child can build a tower of 6 to 7 cubes. When three years old, children can easily place small objects in a small opening and copy a circle. In four years, children can cut out a picture using scissors.

An adolescent or adult can develop new motor skills. A newcomer to a 100 m short race will become more experienced after day-after-day practice. Some players even can reach an extraordinary level. The average high school athlete kid (football player or basketball player) may run 100 meters in approximately 12–13 seconds. A high school boy who does no sports would likely be around 14–15 seconds. Now, the Olympic record for the men's 100 m is 9.58 seconds (by Usain Bolt in 2018).

Patients with motor deficits can also experience recovery. Motor function of patients with stroke or cerebral palsy can regain the motor ability to various extents.

Do these phenomena share a common essence for motor skill development? In other words, what is the core element for acquiring motor skills across these fields? For stroke rehabilitation, the facilitation model argued that the movement pattern was the element of movement, and we thus need to correct abnormal movement patterns to improve the motor function of stroke patients. The motor relearning program, developed by Carr and Shepherd, considered biomedical elements as the key factor of normal movements, and medical professionals should train stroke patients to master these elements. In the field of sports training, muscle strength, durability, coordination and flexibility often constitute basic components of exercise.

To perform whatever types of movement, it needs muscle activities to move trunks and limbs. Muscle contractions are driven by the central nervous system (CNS). CNS activates muscles to generate suitable forces, which move the body along the right trajectory with the right timing. It is a crucial ability to exert suitable muscle force for successfully performing a motor action. The motor performance of the action is the manifestation of exerted muscular force, which can be used to assess the quality of the movement. The essence of developing motor skills is to **learn the right way to exert muscle force when performing a motor task**, that is, a rational force-exerting mode. A rational force-exerting mode drives efficient muscular activities to perform body movements.

Here is an example of a rational force-exerting mode. Hitting a tennis forehand is a common technique. To produce a high-level performance of the forehand drive, different professional tennis players move their wrist to a consistent angular position (wrist hyperextension) at impact during repeated hits though wrist angular velocity near impact is not highly consistent [6, 7]. Such a wrist angular position at impact consistently appears in professional tennis players and thus can be called a "rational" position. The muscle activity to achieve this position is driven by a rational force-exerting mode under the specific situation (i.e., hitting a tennis forehand).

Let's take another example from common people. Upward reaching in shoulder flexion and sideward reaching in shoulder abduction involve in different spatial-temporal patterns of the pectoralis major and serratus anterior muscle in healthy adults [8]. A given spatial-temporal pattern for the corresponding reaching type (upward or sideward) is driven by the rational force-exerting mode of the action [9].

The normal spatial-temporal changes in EMG signals [10] represent a rational force-exerting mode. A rational force-exerting mode is the subjective "feeling" or maneuver by which a motor action is driven properly and efficiently, e.g., pushing the heel down to the floor when training leg extensors [11]. This is a skill often successfully activating extensors in lower limbs, whereas it may not be effective to achieve the same goal by focusing on contracting the leg extensors. Another example is to activate the serratus anterior by using push-ups plus simultaneously arching the interscapular region [12], rather than focusing on where the muscle lies and trying to contract it. The "draw-in" maneuver [13] is also an example, which is often used to activate the transversus abdominis muscle; this maneuver is performed by drawing in the lower abdomen or navel toward the spine. Notably, all these force-exerting modes do not let the subject/patient pay attention to the primary movers. Instead, the subjects need to look for and experience a mode by which the force is exerted properly.

For a given motor action, a rational force-exerting mode is often learned intentionally, e.g., by professional training in athletes (for hitting a tennis forehand) or through everyday practice (for an infant learning to walk). Through learning and feedback, a rational force-exerting mode may be built.

Movement pattern and force-exerting mode

A force-exerting mode is different from a movement pattern or a biomechanical component.

Until now, movement pattern is a term frequently used in the literature and clinical practice in stroke rehabilitation. Brunnstrom observed stereotyped movement patterns (synergies) in adult patients with hemiplegia and described four basic limb synergies, flexor synergy of the upper limb, extensor synergy of the upper limb, flexor synergy of the lower limb, and extensor synergy of the lower limb. The movement patterns consist either of a gross flexor movement or a gross extensor movement. A movement pattern indicates a synergy caused by contractions of a group of muscles, e.g., the basic limb synergies introduced by Brunnstrom [14]:

> The flexor synergy of the upper limb consists of retraction and/or elevation of the shoulder girdle, external rotation of the shoulder, abduction of the shoulder, supination of the forearm, and flexion of the elbow, whereas the extensor synergy of the upper limb consists of protraction of the shoulder girdle, internal rotation of the shoulder, adduction of the shoulder, pronation of the forearm, and extension of the elbow.
>
> Similarly, the flexor synergy of the lower limb consists of abduction and external rotation of the ankle, flexion of the hip, flexion of the knee, dorsiflexion and eversion of the ankle, and dorsiflexion of the toes, and the extensor synergy of the lower limb consists of adduction and internal rotation of the hip, extension of the hip, extension of the knee, plantar flexion and inversion of the ankle, and plantar flexion of the toes (great toe may extend).

These synergies are used in Brunnstorm's staging of motor function recovery and the Fugl-Meyer assessment. These patterns are called synergies since the muscles activated in the movement are firmly linked together. For example, most or all components a flexor synergy of the upper limb appears when the patient lifts his/her paralyzed arm. Variations do exist across different patients, e.g., some may demonstrate flexion of the wrist but some may not. However, for a given individual, the flexor synergy is very similar if the patient is examined several times in the same manner.

The basic limb synergies were considered to be "primary movement patterns" controlled by the spinal cord, and in healthy adults, the primary movement patterns were modified such that components of these patterns were rearranged by higher centers to drive normal movements.

Whether evoked by reflexes or performed voluntarily, the patient can only contract the participated muscles in the same manner (spatial trajectory and timing) in a flexor synergy or an extensor synergy but is unable to recruit muscles to move a single joint or recruit these same muscles to perform different movement combinations such as the abduction of the shoulder (a component of flexor synergy) with simultaneous elbow extension (a component of extensor synergy).

Such stereotyped movement patterns (synergies) were explained as follows. The central nervous system control skeletal muscles on three levels. The lowest centers output only a few "most automatic" movements, that is, several movement combinations (movement patterns or synergies), but cannot control individual muscle contractions. The middle level controls more voluntary, "less automatic" movements, and the highest level can master muscle activities in "most numerous and most voluntary" movement combinations. It was postulated that due to brain lesions, stroke patients relied mainly on the lowest motor centers and thus could only perform relatively automatic movements, that is, the stereotyped synergies.

Brunnstrom pointed out that the flexion reflex reported by Sherrington, the withdrawal reflex of normal people reported by Hagbarth, and the flexor synergy of the lower limb in hemiplegia patients were (almost) identical movement patterns. She thus concluded that the basic limb synergies of hemiplegia patients were "primitive spinal cord patterns". In a normal person, the spinal cord, as the lowest center, was controlled by higher centers, and therefore components of the basic synergies were rearranged to generate normal motor behavior. After stroke, the primitive, stereotyped movement patterns reappear in stroke patients due to the damaged CNS.

This is a common assumption accepted by all developers of facilitation techniques: since the CNS was thought to control movement patterns, and lesions of the CNS would lead to abnormal patterns of movement, the treatment therefore should focus on suppressing pathological movement patterns or using the pathological movement patterns to restore normal patterns. This is a huge difference from the former "muscle reeducation" concept, which focused on treating individual muscles.

The concept of movement patterns and related facilitation techniques are then applied in clinical practice for decades. However, Gordon argued that it was an oversimplified concept that the brain controls movement but not muscle. The movement patterns are not driven only by wired-in circuits in the lower centers of the CNS. Instead, the interaction between the CNS and the environment leads to the so-called basic limb synergies [5]. The basic limb synergies are stereotyped since the damaged CNS produces abnormal motor outputs, which cannot overcome the limits in the environment (e.g., gravity). As a prominent feature/contribution, the biomechanical analysis is thus always applied in the proposed "motor control model" in the motor relearning program (MRP) [11].

The motor relearning program considers motor actions of healthy people and stroke patients as voluntary movements controlled by the CNS (rather than a combination of reflexes) and influenced by biological features of the muscle and biomechanical factors. The examples of biological features of the muscle include 1) the force generated during a single maximal isometric contraction is determined by the physiological cross-sectional area of a muscle, and 2) a muscle can produce its greatest force in a length where an optimal overlap occurs between the muscle contractile elements (actin and myosin filaments) resulting in a maximum number of cross-bridges. One example of biomechanical factors is that reaching movement can be achieved more easily in the supine position than in the upright position due to less influence of gravity on the movers of the moving arm. This biomechanical advantage of performing reaching in supine is thus used in training upper limb functions and a motor assessment instrument (i.e., the motor assessment scale, MAS).

Another feature of the motor relearning program (and related concepts/approaches) is that the motor training should focus on task-oriented voluntary motor control rather than meaningless movements evoked by reflexes.

Do muscles contract together to form movement patterns?

As introduced previously, the flexion reflex, the withdrawal reflex of healthy people, and the flexor synergy of the lower limb in hemiplegia patients present almost identical movement patterns and thus Brunnstrom considered the basic limb synergies of hemiplegia patients as primitive spinal cord patterns. Then, does the CNS activate muscles separately or together when performing a motor action?

Notably, the well-known upside-down humanoid figure in M1 (the representation of the foot and leg is medial but the arm, face, and mouth areas are more lateral) does not imply that a given part of the motor map separately controls a corresponding body part. The motor map in M1 is not a point-to-point representation of the body. Instead, one motor neuron in M1 controls several different (adjacent) muscles, and one muscle receives projections from several adjacent motor neurons in M1. For example, the cortical motor neurons controlling a single hand muscle, e.g., the adductor pollicis, abductor pollicis longus, or extensor digitorum longus, are widely distributed throughout the arm motor map in M1. Thus, there is a widespread overlap of the distribution of motor neurons projecting to different hand muscles, e.g., the representation areas of the adductor pollicis, abductor pollicis longus, and extensor digitorum longus in M1 overlap [10]. Such overlap implies that coactivation of adjacent muscles occurs when performing a motor action by using one of these muscles and it can be hardly achieved to only activate a single muscle.

However, these small scopes of coactivations do not result in the basic synergies because movements driven by such coactivations are not stereotyped. The complexity of firing patterns of motor neurons [10] makes the coactivation of several nearby muscles produce various motor actions in healthy people. Even the seemingly stereotyped coactivations of leg flexors/extensors, i.e., the basic patterns of human walking, are summations controlled by many small modules in the spinal cord rather than controlled by a big, indivisible single low-level spinal center [15].

In comparison with those in healthy people, most examined wrist muscles in stroke patients exhibit simpler bell-like shapes that present the inability to timely activate muscles, unnecessary long duration of high-level activations, and coactivation of agonist and antagonistic muscles. Such abnormal EMG spatial-temporal changes are accompanied by weak, slow, inaccurate, and discoordinated movements. These abnormal motor behaviors and related EMG changes are often attributed to a deficiency in selective control capabilities after CNS injuries.

The deficiency in selective control capabilities is a result of the "overflow" mechanism. When motor actions are performed by healthy adults, excitatory and inhibitory commands can precisely reach their respective targets (e.g., motor neurons in M1 or the spinal cord) and thus the intensity of nerve impulses to drive muscles can be well controlled. After CNS lesions, the excitatory and inhibitory commands are unable to reach the proper target cells. The intensity of nerve impulses is then increased to improve the intensity of impulses and is sent broadly to increase the possibility to activate target neurons. Compared to the normal condition, it is an overflow out of the normal route and intensity of signal transmission. Selectivity in normal conditions is then disrupted by the overflow, which results in abnormal coactivation of the adjacent muscles in the limb, that is, the basic limb synergies.

To overcome the overflow and resulted basic limb synergies, target motor neurons should be precisely and sufficiently activated, and timely rational inhibition should be achieved. These may be achieved by using a rational force-exerting mode to perform carefully-set motor actions in proper contexts.

A rational force-exerting mode should be built as early as possible

The improper movement patterns repetitively used by stroke patients, i.e., the misuse syndrome, may also be found in other diseases [16, 17].

Essentially, the improper movement patterns are visible manifestations of irrational mode to exert muscle force to complete motor actions, including the jerky, unsmooth, stereotyped spatial trajectory of movements representing poor motor control (e.g., timing and coordination) of involved muscles.

A repetitively occurring behavior leads to the long-term potentiation (LTP), a persistent strengthening of synapses as a result of recent patterns of activities. This is a long-lasting imprint in the CNS that is hard to be changed even for a healthy person, not to mention for a stroke patient with brain lesions that hinders the plasticity of the CNS. An intentionally/unintentionally learned, misused movement pattern, and its corresponding poor force-exerting mode, is often difficult to be corrected and thus should be avoided at the beginning of motor training. For example, many stroke patients fail to activate the serratus anterior muscle when they begin to move the affected arm, and they thus lose the proper scapulohumeral rhythm (also called glenohumeral rhythm), the kinematic interaction between the scapula and the humerus during shoulder movements. Such patients are often unable to activate the serratus anterior properly long after the onset of stroke, which causes shoulder dysfunction and shoulder pain.

The brain and brainstem emit tonic excitatory impulses to the spinal cord, which maintain the normal level of excitation in spinal motor neurons. An acute brain/brainstem lesion interrupts the descending impulses and thus results in a temporary "spinal shock". During the period of the spinal shock, the patient exhibits flaccid paralysis and weakened/disappeared spinal myotatic reflexes. The spinal shock is the flaccid stage in the Brunnstorm's staging. Under most conditions, this state is replaced later by spasticity. However, spasticity and paralysis may appear together, or spinal reflexes may be retained but the limbs remain flaccid in some patients [18].

For stroke patients, the serratus anterior activity is the key component for the rational force-exerting mode of the upper limb movements. The training of the serratus anterior can be started after the early-stage activities of the pectoralis major are found. In this period, all shoulder girdle muscles are weak or have no voluntary contractions and thus the synergies have not been developed. When the arm is perpendicular to the bed in a supine position, assisted reaching is often an effective practice to elicit activities of the serratus anterior. By using surface EMG or ultrasound, weak voluntary muscle contractions at the very early stage can be detected.

Performing this motor action needs proper activations of shoulder flexors, the serratus anterior, and elbow extensors, as well as maintained balance between the internal rotation and external rotation of the shoulder joint and between the pronation and supination of the forearm. This motor action underlies many functional activities of the upper extremities and thus is crucial in the upper limb function training.

A subject can protract or laterally rotate the scapula efficiently and smoothly by properly contracting the serratus anterior. Additionally, the patients may avoid suffering a secondary shoulder impingement syndrome when a rational force-exerting mode of the serratus anterior is developed. The acquired rational force-exerting mode may also migrate to the learning process of other muscles and related motor actions.

Training key motor skills

Extending from the task-oriented concept, motor training should focus on a series of contents that focus on improving key motor skills with practical values, rather than taking efforts to practice a variety of skills less important.

Two key motor functions are crucial for activities of daily living (ADL) and quality of life (QOL), that is, reaching and walking. Reaching is a motor action that a hand moves forward or sideways towards a target, with an extending elbow and the flexion of the shoulder (glenohumeral) joint. Shoulder flexion muscles, the serratus anterior, and elbow and wrist extensors are primary movers of a reaching action, and the balance between the internal rotation and external rotation of the shoulder joint and between the pronation and supination of the forearm should be maintained. These components of reaching underlie arm movements in front of the body, such as hand/arm movements during feeding, taking/putting down things, and holding and manipulating smartphones. Reaching forward is more closely related to function and is more difficult to be well controlled by stroke patients in comparison with reaching sideways.

Hence, reaching forward and walking should be two core elements of motor training in stroke patients. Training the two elements has higher priority in comparison with other motor skills. Since it may take much effort and time to acquire a motor skill for stroke patients, training the key contents is efficient and productive.

Algorithm for training forward reaching

1) Test whether the patients can voluntarily adduct the shoulder (glenohumeral) joint in the supine position (pectoralis major), which is often the first voluntary movement of the affected upper limb and is usually much easier to be activated than the serratus anterior.

2) Activate the serratus anterior muscle through forward reaching, i.e., reaching towards the ceiling. The arm is placed in a position perpendicular to the bed (i.e., forward flexion of the shoulder joint) in a supine position with the elbow extended and wrist slightly extended; assistance is often needed to help the patient maintain the position. See whether the shoulder protraction appears. The proper action of the shoulder protraction looks like extending a retractable antenna mast section by section, rather than moving the shoulder as a whole. A slight resistance may be applied around the arm or wrist to guide the direction of the movement. Avoid improper alignment such as internal rotation of the shoulder joint or pronation of the forearm. Surface EMG or ultrasound is helpful to detect mild muscle contractions at the very early stage.

3) Let the patient hold the perpendicular position after reaching, and gradually decrease the assistance. A successful holding needs a better capacity to control shoulder girdle muscles and elbow extensors than reaching. Train isometric, eccentric, and concentric contractions of the shoulder protraction movers; motor actions should be performed smoothly at a relatively uniform speed, and the appearance of extending a retractable antenna mast should always to monitored.

4) Slight lower the arm (reduce the shoulder flexion angle), and exercise the reaching forward action along the direction of the long axis of the arm. Maintain the proper alignment. Exercise position-holding when reaching forward can be achieved. Try to move the arm back to the perpendicular position.

5) Gradually reduce the shoulder flexion angle and repeat exercises in the previous step, until the patient can lower the arm to the bed and lift it to the perpendicular position smoothly with a proper alignment and a relatively low speed (e.g., 4-5 s from zero to 90 degrees).

6) In a sitting position, hold the arm in the 80-90 degrees of shoulder forward flexion. Exercise reaching forward. After the patient can perform the action with a rational mode, exercise position-holding, and practice with a gradually lowered arm.

The above steps mainly focus on movers of the shoulder protraction and flexion and elbow extensors. These muscles are not the strongest ones of the arm and should girdle but play key roles in reaching forward. Other exercises to train these muscles and other muscles may be helpful, whereas the algorithm presents the core contents.

Algorithm for training walking

1) Exercise bridging in the supine position to strengthen hip and trunk extensors. Avoid improper alignments such as pelvic tilt or an excessive forward curve of the lumbar spine. Press down the anterior superior iliac spine, or let the patient push the heel down to the bed may activate muscle contractions. Once bridging on both feet can be successfully performed,

exercise bridging only on the affected foot using the training action introduced by Carr et al [11]. Maintaining the sitting position in the bed as early as possible to improve trunk control.

2) Exercise standing when a good sitting position can be held and the hip joint can be fully extended and the position can be maintained with a proper alignment. A knee immobilizer and a solid ankle-foot orthosis are often needed.

3) A lateral bridging exercise may be used to strengthen hip abductors, which is important in standing and walking.

4) Standing on the affected foot when placing the other foot on a step. Maintain a proper alignment. Slightly change the degree of the knee joint (from zero to 15 degrees) of the affected leg during standing exercise. This position-hold exercise is very effective to strengthen leg extensors, including the gluteus maximus, quadratus femoris, gastrocnemius, and soleus.

5) Practice walking forward after a safe standing is achieved. A knee immobilizer and a solid ankle-foot orthosis can be helpful at the early stage. Parallel bars or a body weight support system can be used in weak patients. Many patients may have not enough potential to regain a (nearly) normal gait, and it is hard to see the effect of training leg flexors (hip and knee flexors, and ankle dorsiflexors) on gait improvement although relevant specific techniques exist.

A lateral bridging exercise may be used to strengthen hip abductors in any stage if the proper pelvic alignment cannot be achieved or maintained.

Note that the gastrocnemius and soleus are important for knee control during standing and walking. A solid ankle-foot orthosis may partially replace some functions of the muscles.

Safe standing is a prerequisite for walking exercise. And the capacity to maintain a proper sitting position is the prerequisite for standing. A treadmill or walking robotic may be helpful but is not indispensable for walking training. Walking with a (nearly) normal rhythm and pattern cannot be achieved in many stroke patients. Under such conditions, good control of the trunk and leg extensors and hip abductors are crucial to standing and walking safely. The steps introduced above train very basic elements for walking. At the early stage, many training contents such as supine-to-sit, sitting balance, sit-to-stand transition, and hip flexor exercise in supine should be skipped and the exercise should focus on standing and walking. Early-emerging voluntary walking may facilitate further gait recovery, and a walkable patient is more likely to learn supine-to-sit, sit-to-stand transition, and hip flexion.

Summary

Here, a rational force-exerting mode is proposed as a basic principle during motor training in stroke patients. In healthy adults, the CNS drives a simple motor action by activating a number of adjacent muscles due to lacking a one-on-one relationship between cortical motor neurons and muscles. Normal CNS structure and function provide high flexibility to use such coactivations to perform various types of skillful movements. Movements under normal motor control exhibit coordinated spatial-temporal relationship among activations of all involved muscles and is thus highly flexible and efficient. Patients with lesions in the CNS lose such fine-grained capacity for motor control, which is sometimes considered a deficiency in selective control capabilities, i.e., the inability to activate some muscle (s) when inhibiting other muscles. All these abnormalities in motor control result in abnormal motor performance in stroke patients, so-called stereotyped movement patterns such as the flexor/extensor synergies of the upper or lower limbs.

The force-exerting mode is a "deeper" concept than movement patterns and biomechanical components. Movement patterns are often used to describe the appearance or performance of motor actions. Hemiplegia patients present stereotyped movement patterns (synergies); as motor functions are improved, more selected movements appear. In the motor relearning program, biomechanical components are introduced as essential parts to complete motor actions. Here, note that all voluntary movements are driven by muscle forces. Thus, it is the force-exerting mode that influences movement patterns. On the other hand, a biomechanical component can be completed by a rational (if a motor action is performed smoothly, coordinated, and efficiently) or irrational force-exerting mode. If a patient can complete a biomechanical component but in an uncoordinated and unsmooth manner, we consider that the adopted force-exerting mode is not rational.

A specific task orienting a motor action provides a practical value (and therefore motivation) to the action. To perform a motor action, a subject needs to apply a mode to exert force. The adopted force-exerting mode, whether rational/efficient or not, may be intentional or unintentional. A high-level athlete can use the most rational/efficient way to drive muscles to complete difficult motor actions, whereas a stroke patient often performs a motor action with discoordinated, awkward, and stereotyped movement patterns driven by a poor mode to exert force.

A rational force-exerting mode has better be trained at the very early stage after stroke onset. Otherwise, the misuse syndrome is likely to be developed and is often hard to be corrected. The developed poor force-exerting mode drives those typical movement patterns observed in stroke patients and hinders the rational force-exerting mode.

Training the rational force-exerting mode is recommended during motor rehabilitation of two key motor skills, reaching forward and walking. Each of them has a corresponding algorithm. Specific techniques and requirements are needed to develop a rational force-exerting mode.

Whether a motor action is driven by a rational force-exerting mode, the patient presents a higher-level performance. For example, if the patient cannot fully extend the hip joint, a rational force-exerting mode (e.g., pushing the heel down to the floor) may help the subject complete the full range of extension. This is a from-weak-to-strong or develop-from-nothing process. Under such conditions, the rational force-exerting mode is used to initiate or enhance muscle contractions. Another type of rational force-exerting mode is to generate smooth, coordinated, unstiffened, and relatively slow movements with the proper alignment. This may be acquired by training the motion action/muscles with specific techniques including various combinations of eccentric, concentric, and isometric contractions, moving with slow and uniform speeds, and building the proper "experience" of moving. The proper experience of moving is similar to "interoception", that is, feeling sensations from the inside of the body [19, 20]. Under such conditions, the rational force-exerting mode is used to build skills to manipulate muscle contractions, a stage often later than the initiation and enhancement, though building skills should often be combined with the enhancement (strengthen muscles). For some patients with high selective movement control (e.g., those in Brunnstorm's 5th stage), high-level dexterity, explosive force, and other advanced properties of the force-exerting mode may be needed.

References

[1] Allan HR, Brown RH. Adams and Victor's Principles of Neurology. 2005. 8th ed. New York. McGraw-Hill. 660-746.

[2] Stinear CM. Prediction of motor recovery after stroke: advances in biomarkers. Lancet Neurol. 2017； 16: 826-836.

[3] Stinear CM, Byblow WD, Ackerley SJ, Smith MC, Borges VM, Barber PA. Proportional Motor Recovery After Stroke: Implications for Trial Design. Stroke. 2017； 48: 795-798.

[4] Neumann DA. Polio: its impact on the people of the United States and the emerging profession of physical therapy. J Orthop Sports Phys Ther. 2004； 34: 479-92.

[5] Gordon J. Assumptions underlying physical therapy intervention: theoretical and historical approaches. In: Carr JH, Shepherd R eds. Movement Science: Foundations for Physical Therapy in Rehabilitation. 1987. Rockville, MD. Aspen Publishers Inc. 1–30.

[6] Elliott B. Biomechanics and tennis. Br J Sports Med. 2006； 40: 392-6.

[7] Knudson D. Intrasubject Variability of Upper Extremity Angular Kinematics in the Tennis Forehand Drive. International Journal of Sport Biomechanics. 1990； 6: 415.

[8] Hiengkaew V, Wichaiwong K, Chaiyakul S, Deesin A. Concerning the pectoralis major in active reaching exercise. Electromyogr Clin Neurophysiol. 2003； 43: 157-63.

[9] Basmaijan JV, De Luca CJ. Muscles alive. 1985. 265-289.

[10] Rizzolatti G, Kalaska JF. Voluntary Movement: The Primary Motor Cortex. In: Kandel ER, Schwartz JH, Jessell TM, Siegelbaum SA, Hudspeth AJ eds. Principles of Neural Science. 2013. London. McGraw-Hill. 835-864.

[11] Janet HC, Roberta BS. A Motor Relearning Programme for Stroke. 1987. 2nd. Rockville, USA. Aspen Publishers.

[12] Kirkesola G. Neurac – a new treatment method for long-term musculoskeletal pain. Fysioterapeuten. 2009； 76: 16-25.

[13] Sapsford RR, Hodges PW, Richardson CA, Cooper DH, Markwell SJ, Jull GA. Co-activation of the abdominal and pelvic floor muscles during voluntary exercises. Neurourol Urodyn. 2001； 20: 31-42.

[14] Brunnstrom S. Movement Therapy in Hemiplegia: a Neurophysiological Approach. 1982. 1st. Virginia, USA. Harper & Row, Publishers, Inc. 1-192.

[15] Hägglund M, Dougherty KJ, Borgius L, Itohara S, Iwasato T, Kiehn O. Optogenetic dissection reveals multiple rhythmogenic modules underlying locomotion. Proc Natl Acad Sci U S A. 2013； 110: 11589-94.

[16] Clarke J. Organizing the approach to musculoskeletal misuse syndrome. Nurse Pract. 2001; 26: 11-5, 19-25.

[17] Pan R, Zhou M, Cai H, et al. A randomized controlled trial of a modified wheelchair arm-support to reduce shoulder pain in stroke patients. Clin Rehabil. 2018; 32: 37-47.

[18] Allan HR, Brown RH. Adams and Victor's Principles of Neurology. 2005. 8th ed. New York. McGraw-Hill. 53-58.

[19] Craig AD. Interoception: the sense of the physiological condition of the body. Curr Opin Neurobiol. 2003; 13: 500-5.

[20] Craig AD. How do you feel? Interoception: the sense of the physiological condition of the body. Nat Rev Neurosci. 2002; 3: 655-66.

Q AND A FOR MOTOR SKILL TRAINING IN STROKE PATIENTS

What is selective motor control?

Selective motor control is considered as an ability to activate/contract a given muscle separately, i.e., without evoking undesired movement driven by other muscles. Broadly speaking, selective motor control represents the ability of the CNS to choose a target, a target level, or a time window, that is, to activate a muscle/a group of muscles, to activate muscle contractions to a certain level, or to maintain the desired activation level in a given period. The selective control is therefore the cornerstone of normal motor behavior, in contrast with the synergies (i.e., stereotyped movement patterns).

Since there is no point-to-point correspondence between the motor neurons in M1 and the skeletal muscles, so-called "selective" motor control does not imply that M1 can selectively activate a single muscle (or a group of muscles with very similar functions) by activating a group of adjacent M1 motor neurons. For example, many arm muscles exhibit overlapped representation areas in M1, and thus shoulder muscles are activated when moving the wrist whereas wrist muscles are activated when moving the shoulder. That is, many arm muscles are activated simultaneously when a single joint movement is performed, even though some of these muscles are not adjacent to the moved joint [1].

From this point of view, a "mini" movement pattern exists for every single joint movement. Even for a single joint movement, a person with a normal level of motor control does not selectively activate a single muscle but only selectively activates the primary mover more intensively than a number of nearby muscles.

Despite all this, specifically combined activations in chosen muscles can be achieved, e.g., shoulder protraction and flexion, and elbow extension can be driven simultaneously to complete functional motor actions. This type of motor action is not a result of recombining broken "basic synergies" but can be directly formed by arranging activities of adjacent muscles.

What is the cause of the "basic synergies"?

The basic synergies (several stereotyped movement patterns) are the results of CNS lesions after stroke, muscle biological and biomechanical factors, constraints from the environment (mainly the impact of gravity), and the irrational force-exerting mode.

The basic synergies are not solely attributed to neurophysiological issues, e.g., only driven by wired-in circuits in the CNS, and thus may be modified by arranging the above-listed factors.

Hemiplegia patients often move limbs in a hurried and reckless manner partially influenced by the impression that he/she can control their limb movements easily before the disease onset. This manner is a typical irrational force-exerting mode after stroke. Since ***the emotion-motivation system in the CNS presents tight connections with the motor system***, a special training protocol for developing a rational force-exerting mode is crucial for better motor control. A developed rational force-exerting mode may also help the patient to avoid the overflow effect.

The muscle biological and biomechanical impacts involve factors such as the force-length relationship of a muscle (e.g., in which length a muscle can perform maximum contraction), the relation between the maximum force and the cross-sectional area of a muscle, the Leverage mechanism, and viscoelastic properties of muscles and other adjacent soft tissues (e.g., contractures).

What is the "overflow" effect?

In healthy adults, excitatory commands are accurately sent to target motor neurons in the cortex and then in the spinal cord, so dost inhibitory commands. Due to interruption of the pathway after CNS lesions, these commands cannot reach the proper target motor neurons. A common response is to take more effort to complete the motor action, which generates stronger excitatory commands and these commands are sent to a broader scope of motor neurons. This is called the "overflow" (out of the normal route of command passing). As a result, the agonist, antagonist, synergist of a motor action, and even those muscles uninvolved under normal conditions are activated. The stronger excitatory commands also lead to temporal derangement of muscle activations.

The overflow is a result of lacking selectivity and should be avoided or overcome during motor training when building a ration force-exerting mode. Two core features of a ration force-exerting mode are to precisely activate the target muscle(s) and to use an effort without exceeding the needs of the motor action ("using the smallest force"). The first feature aims to train selectivity, and the second feature aims to enhance the controlling capacity to modulate the intensity of applied efforts. Also note adopting a constant and relatively slow speed at the early stage of motor training, which benefits maintaining a smooth movement and thus trains coordination.

The overflow effect may be useful when a weak muscle needs to be activated. When applying resistance on the upper arm, performing reaching forward may elicit the overflow effect: enhanced activity in the serratus anterior driving the shoulder protraction can be overflowed to elbow extensors. Also, see the answer on "evoke ankle dorsiflexion": resist voluntary flexion of the hip or knee to activate ankle flexors. This is an example of overflow. Similar techniques are used in Brunnstrom and PNF training contents. Be careful to use the overflow effect since it is easy to develop an improper force-exerting mode.

How is "the smallest force" determined?

When a healthy adult reaches forward to touch a push button, a number of muscles are activated. The smallest force is the minimum contracting intensity of the agonists (e.g., the serratus anterior, shoulder flexors, and elbow extensors) with which the proper alignment is achieved at a constant and relatively slow speed. Practically, a smooth, coordinated, unstiffened, and relatively slow movement with a proper alignment indicates the subject uses the smallest force to complete that task.

The smallest force is a method to train the selectivity of motor control. When this force-exerting mode can be repeatedly achieved, exercise to enhance muscle strength can be considered.

Why use a constant and relatively slow speed?

At a constant and relatively slow speed, the quality of a motor action is easy to be observed. The patient is more likely to "experience" the selective activation of a given muscle (or its effect). Such a speed is also easier for the patient to adjust if the motor performance is less than expected.

Should the constant and slow speed be used throughout the training?

No. When a force-exerting mode is built and the proper movement pattern can be seen, the patient may be trained to gradually increase the speed of a motor action (and enhance the strength of the agonists). A proper alignment should always be maintained.

However, note that a faster speed is very likely to evoke overflow effects and obstruct the observation of deficits in motor performance.

How to selectively enhance muscle strength?

Some specially designed motor actions may be used, combined with vibration/electrical stimulation or other facilitation techniques. For example, practice pushing down the hand when taking weight through the affected arm on the lateral side or front of the body, in a sitting or standing position with a fully extended elbow. Avoid excessive internal rotation of the shoulder joint and pronation of the forearm. This is a variation of the push-up exercises and can activate the serratus anterior, shoulder flexors, and elbow extensors. Sometimes it is more effective than reaching forward. It is a closed-kinetic-chain exercise combined with weight bearing (or resistance training). This type of exercise is very effective to activate muscles (see the Neurac technique [2] for details)

The closed-kinetic-chain exercise combined with weight-bearing/ resistance-training and peripheral sensory inputs often evokes strong muscle activations. Thus, it is a good approach to initiate or enhance muscle contractions.

When performing strength training, the patients should exhibit a “smooth” movement when enough force is generated. That is, the muscle force is smoothly “transferred” along the limb but not “stuck” somewhere. Otherwise, the force-exerting mode is not rational.

What are peripheral facilitation and central facilitation?

As introduced by Sherrington, facilitation or inhibition is the process in which the excitability of a group of neurons is enhanced or weakened via temporal/spatial summations of synaptic potentials. In addition to those well-known peripherally applied sensory inputs by various facilitation techniques, central factors may facilitate motor outputs and enhance stronger muscle activities. One example is the role of the CNS emotional/motivation system in motor control: a very “decisive” or “inspiring” verbal instruction can evoke stronger muscle activities than a “dull” verbal command. Additionally, a sequential facilitation technique may be applied: if the patient cannot flex fingers at the beginning of a treatment session, the shoulder adductors and then elbow and wrist flexors can be evoked and strengthened. Afterwards, the voluntary movement of finger flexors may be evoked. This phenomenon can be explained by the overlap of muscle representation areas in M1 (and other cortical motor areas). Via these overlaps, voluntary movements of one end of a limb may be evoked by sequentially evoking muscle contractions in other parts of the limb.

The classical Brunnstrom and PNF techniques use resistance training together with concurrent voluntary efforts, which summits peripheral and central mechanisms to elicit strong muscle coactivations (possibly at the cost of losing selectivity).

What are the methods to evoke ankle dorsiflexion?

Ankle dorsiflexion is driven by the tibialis anterior, extensor hallucis longus, extensor digitorum longus, and peroneous tertius. The actions of the tibialis anterior and extensor hallucis longus are ankle dorsiflexion with simultaneous ankle/foot inversion. Only the extensor digitorum longus and peroneous tertius can dorsiflex the ankle with simultaneous ankle eversion. Thus, the ankle dorsiflexion without (excessive) inversion can only be achieved when the extensor digitorum longus and peroneous tertius are well activated. Note that the Peroneous brevis and Peroneous longus evert the ankle only during ankle plantarflexion; these muscles are elongated when the ankle is dorsiflexed.

A recess lies between the lateral malleolus and the peroneal trochlea of the calcaneus, which is the opening of the sinus tarsi. Place the index finger on the anterior border of the lateral malleolus, move the finger inferiorly toward the sole of the foot, and then it will slide into the recess. In some subjects, a prominent muscle belly of the extensor digitorum brevis may be touched in the recess.

Pressing downward the soft tissue in the recess may evoke ankle dorsiflexion in the affected side in some patients when the patient lies supine and flex the affected hip and knee joints. In some patients, ankle dorsiflexion with eversion can be seen. If ankle dorsiflexion can be evoked, let the patient voluntarily flex the hip, knee, and ankle with the maximum effort, resist such flexions (at the thigh, calf, or dorsum foot), and simultaneously apply the pressing-downward stimulation. Such a combination may evoke stronger ankle dorsiflexion. Afterwards, decrease the external stimuli and let the patient dorsiflex the ankle voluntarily. Once the ankle dorsiflexion can be voluntarily completed, let the patient gradually extend the hip and knee and try to perform ankle dorsiflexion. The methods introduced by Carr et al [3] and Davis [4] may also be used.

If the patient cannot dorsiflex the foot, a solid ankle-foot orthosis may be applied to maintain a rational alignment. Additionally, the solid ankle-foot orthosis may stabilize the knee during standing and walking.

How should the ankle plantarflexion be trained?

Unless the patient has enough dorsiflexion control, strength training of ankle plantar flexors should be carefully applied to avoid spasticity.

During standing, using the affected lower limb bears the body weight is an effective exercise to enhance ankle plantarflexion control. The patient may perform the position-holding exercises first. If the proper alignment can be maintained, changing the knee joint angle in the range of 0°-15° (full extension = 0°) at a constant and relatively slow speed. These exercises also improve the standing control capacity of the lower limb.

As an advanced exercise, the patient places the front half of the affected feet on a stair, with the other foot (entire sole) on the upper stair and the body weight bearing on the affected forefoot. Let the patient lift and lower the heel on the affected side at a relatively slow speed and pause at any point, following the instructions. Concentric, eccentric, and isometric contractions of the ankle plantar flexor are thus exercised. The patient can experience how to control the "push-up" of the forefoot against the surface of the stair step to complete the movements.

What roles do ankle plantarflexion muscles play in standing and walking?

An important issue is ankle plantarflexion muscles play a key role in maintaining knee extension during standing and walking. The knee extension is not solely controlled by the knee extensor, i.e., the quadriceps femoris. Thus, exercises to enhance muscle force of ankle plantarflexion muscles should be performed when a stroke patient presents a deficit of 0°-15° knee extension control.

What are the key points when training a rational force-exerting mode?

There are two situations, 1) initiate/enhance muscle contractions and 2) fine-grained motor control training.

When a motor action cannot be voluntarily performed by the patient, or the patient can only exert very weak forces to drive the motor action, "guiding" techniques can be used to initiate/enhance muscle contractions.

When the motor action can be completed repeatedly but is unsmooth, stiff, and/or discoordinated to some extent, the "quality" of the movement should be improved. In this situation, a rational force-exerting mode is learned by exercising specific types of motor actions. Let the patient exactly follow the verbal instructions to perform the motor actions. Especially, initiate the movement after the verbal command is given. Following the required speed (possibly indicated by the therapist), maintain a proper alignment, or keep making adjustments towards a proper alignment. Once an expected mode is built when performing a motor action, gradually change the range of motion, moving speed, and types of muscle contractions (isometric, eccentric, and concentric) to provide variations.

What is the "guiding technique"?

Here are several examples:

Train reaching forward in a supine position, and resistance is applied at the arm or wrist to "guide" the movement. Some patients may immediately find a way to complete shoulder protraction via the contraction of the serratus anterior.

Let the patient take weight through the affected arm in front of the body in a sitting position with the elbow fully extended, and push down the hand on the root of the palm to activate the serratus anterior.

Let the patient push the heel down to the floor when practicing single-leg bridging or sitting-to-standing, to activate hip and knee extensors.

For each of these closed-kinetic-chain exercises or resistance exercises (possibly combined with weight-bearing training), a target point is used to generate resistance to "guild" the motor action. By using such a guiding technique, the patient is more likely to find a way to activate the agonist (s) to complete the movement.

Are there any methods to evoke voluntary activities of a completely paralyzed muscle?

Use a specific posture and action listed in the Algorithms. Those biomechanically benefit voluntary motor control and/or have high practical value.

Usually, a muscle is more likely to be activated in its middle length. With actin-myosin binding, the cross-bridge transitions from a weakly bound low-force state to a strongly bound high-force state. The magnitude of muscle force depends on sarcomere length and the overlap between thick and thin filaments, which determines the fraction of cross-bridges. Based on the measured active force-length relationship, the maximum force appears approximately at the middle length of a muscle.

Voluntary contractions of a muscle may be evoked first by using concentric, eccentric, or isometric contractions in different patients.

Electrical stimulation, vibration, presenting resistance, or painful stimulation may be helpful to evoke voluntary muscle contractions.

Verbal commands in an exciting tone are better than dull commands.

The sequential facilitation technique may be applied.

If a muscle contracts as a synergist, it is more likely to contract as an agonist. For example, elbow extensors may not voluntarily contract when being recruited as agonists, but a relatively strong shoulder protraction may accompany contractions of elbow extensors when a forward reaching is exercised.

How should fine-grained motor control training be performed?

Still, use a specific posture and action listed in the Algorithms. Gradually transfer to other postures.

Use a constant, relatively slow speed during movement.

Exactly follow the oral instructions.

Maintain proper alignments.

Practice concentric, eccentric, and isometric contractions for a given muscle.

Practice interruptions and reinitiation during movements

Practice graded contractions, i.e., divided the entire ROM into several parts, and complete the ROM via a "concentric contraction, pause/isometric contraction, concentric contraction,…" and a reverse "eccentric contraction, pause/isometric contraction, eccentric contraction,…" sequence.

How is the rational force-exerting mode explained biomechanically?

At a given speed, a rational force-exerting mode is the one by which a subject completes a motor action along an optimal trajectory, by using a minimum force and a proper alignment. Here, the term "rational" instead of "optimal" is used since the training is designed for ordinary people but not top-level athletes.

A minimum force is a force generated by the agonist(s) and synergist(s) that is just enough to complete the motor action. It is therefore the most "economical" force. Exercising such a minimum force can reduce the "overflow" effect.

Does the nonhemiplegic side provide help for building a rational force-exerting mode?

The exercises (such as those introduced in the "guiding technique") may be performed by the nonhemiplegic side of the patient. After a rational force-exerting mode is acquired on this side, the hemiplegic side may be more likely to learn how to develop the rational mode. This may rely on dense projections across the corpus callosum and strong functional connectivity between homotopic brain regions during unilateral limb movements [5].

Why a rational force-exerting mode should be developed as early as possible?

When learning a new force-exerting mode, new synapses are developed and weak synapses are strengthened. This is a trial-and-error process in which the synaptic connections are weak and changeable.

A developed force-exerting mode and accompanied movement patterns, whether rational or not, form persistent strengthening of synapses (the long-term potentiation, LTP). These "fixed" pathways are hard to be modified due to the limited plasticity of the CNS in stroke patients.

Additionally, a rational force-exerting mode for one motor action may be transferred to other motor actions, and so does the improper mode to exert force to perform a motor action. Thus, it is optional to build a rational force-exerting mode as early as possible.

What is the difference between a motor task and a motor action?

Both are motor actions. A task implies hard or unpleasant work that has to be done whereas an action is a neutral statement, thus here the term "motor action" is preferred.

Training a rational force-exerting mode is performance-based, that is, to determine whether the force-exerting mode is a proper one according to the motor performance. The adopted motor actions are those crucial for ADL and are therefore also task-oriented.

What is the difference between facilitation techniques, task-oriented/biomechanical-analysis-based training (e.g., the motor learning program), and motor skill training based on the rational force-exerting mode?

Conventional facilitation techniques focus on using movement patterns to improve motor function. Normal motor behaviors are considered to be the results of recombined components of several basic movement patterns/synergies.

The motor learning program considers the motor behavior of stroke patients as results caused by mixed reasons, especially biomechanical factors, and biological features of the muscle in addition to the CNS.

The motor performance of the stroke patient is driven by the force-exerting mode. Thus, training the rational force-exerting mode is crucial to developing high-quality motor control in stroke patients.

A motor learning or relearning process is a process to build a rational force-exerting mode. Once a rational force-exerting mode is acquired for a given motor action, the skill can be transferred to other motor actions. Additionally, several key motor actions are chosen to improve the efficiency of motor training.

Why those key motor actions are important?

These motor actions are listed in the Algorithm for training forward reaching and Algorithm for training walking. Reaching forward and walking are two core functions in ADL and therefore have a higher priority in comparison with other motor skills.

Using the hand freely relies on good motor control of the shoulder and arm. Some stroke patients may have not enough motor control capacity to use hemiplegic shoulder and arm but have a much better hand function if effective training were not received. Reaching forward contains the basic motor components of daily-used shoulder and arm movements. Notably, not all stroke patients have the potential to regain good upper limb function. For these patients, walking ability training should be focused on.

Why not exercise sit-to-stand prior to those key motor actions for walking?

Patients with the ability to walk independently can transfer developed motor control ability to many other functions involving trunk and leg participation.

Once a stroke patient walks independently, the ability of sit-to-stand transfer can be easily acquired. On the contrary, a stroke patient who can complete a sit-to-stand transfer may still be difficult to learn walking. Therefore, training functions directly related to walking prior to sit-to-stand is more efficient.

Are rhythmic movements important for recovering walking ability?

Body-weight support treadmill exercises and robotic-assisted training can provide rhythmic bilateral leg movements to simulate normal gait patterns. Compared to gait rhythm, the weight-bearing ability is fundamental for walking safely. This is how the Algorithm for training walking is designed. In the Algorithm, a series of exercises are provided, which focus on developing the weight-bearing ability of the patients.

The patient can walk once the weight-bearing ability is regained, which is not related to how well a rhythmic bilateral leg movement is achieved in a walking-assistance device. However, such instruments can help the patient perform weight-bearing movements at the early stage after stroke onset and thus are helpful.

How should ataxia be treated?

Frenkel's exercises can be used to correct ataxia. Briefly, the patient should practice a series of specific motor actions with a constant and relatively slow speed when the affected upper/lower limb bears slight weights, e.g., by using sandbags. A target point/area/line is provided, and the patient should try to move the limb towards/following the target as exactly as possible. Via the visual feedback of how exactly the target is matched, the patient can learn whether the applied force-exerting mode is rational.

Both proprioceptive and visual inputs benefit coordination. Here, we emphasize that the force-exerting mode should be experienced during weight-bearing training to enhance the processing of proprioceptive inputs; this is *different* from some types of Frenkel's exercises only using visual inputs. Also, note that a constant speed is preferred during movement. Present the speed by moving the arm/hand, which the patient can follow.

In Frenkel's exercises, the training focused on improving coordination but not muscle strength. Thus, fatigue should be avoided. The verbal commands are given via an even, slow voice (rather than using an exciting or inspiring manner for hemiplegia patients to activate the emotional/motivational system). Simple exercises should be performed repeatedly until progress is achieved. Afterwards, more difficult training can be provided. Since whether the target is matched relies on visual inputs, the patient should be in a position to see his/her moving limb and the target.

The first several practice actions can be performed at a faster speed. Once the target is matched, slower speeds can be applied.

When a motor action can be completed at a slow and constant speed, verbal commands to interrupt the movement can be tried, that is, a continual movement is changed into several segments with pauses.

The following exercises are used in patients with ataxia but without or with mild hemiplegia. For patients with moderate hemiplegia and ataxia, training contents listed in the Algorithm for reaching and walking can be used, together with slight weight-bearing, resistance (guiding techniques), or concurrent electrical stimulation to enhance proprioceptive inputs.

Upper limb exercises:

Face a blackboard. Use chalk to change a minus sign to a plus sign.

Copy straight lines, triangles, cubes, circles, and zig-zag lines, or move a finger along such figures.

Exercises in supine:

The patient lies on the bed with a smooth surface along which the feet can easily slide. The head is supported on a pillow so that the patient can see the position of the leg and feet.

1). Flex the hip and knee of one leg, and then slide the heel along the surface of the bed. Return to the starting position by straightening the leg. Repeat the motor action with the other leg. During movements, keep the heel constantly contacting the bed surface. The moving speed and direction should follow the moving hand of the therapist.
2). Flex the hip and knee of one leg. Abduct the flexed hip, and then return (adduct the hip) to the neutral position. Return to the starting position. Repeat the motor action with the other leg. The moving speed and direction should follow the moving hand of the therapist.
3). Perform the above-introduced motor actions, stopping at any point. The moving speed, direction, and pause should follow the moving hand of the therapist.
4). Flex both hips and knees simultaneously, and then perform abduction, adduction, and extension. Stop at any point. Try to complete motor actions symmetrically.
5). Flex/extend two legs alternately at the hips and knees in a bicycling motion.

A constant speed is preferred. Once motor actions are well performed with weight-bearing, the born weight can be reduced or removed.

Exercises of sitting-to-standing:

The patient sits on a chair or PT bed with feet flat on the floor.

1). Draw footprints on the floor. Raise one heel, and then gradually lift the entire foot. Place the foot exactly on the footprint. Alternately repeat the action with two feet.

2). Mark lines on the floor with chalk or other tools. Alternately glide the heel along the line in a forward, backward, left, or right direction.

3). Learn forward to rise from the chair/PT bed and sit again following a counted rhythm (order): at one, flex knees and move feet under the chair/PT bed; at two, flex hip joints and move trunk forward; at three, rise by extending hips and knees. Sit down by reversing the process.

Exercises during standing:

Stand erect with feet 4 to 6 inches apart.

1). Walk forward between two parallel lines 14 inches apart. Place the right foot just inside the right line and the left foot just inside the left line. Try to complete the correct placements.

2). Walk forward. Place each foot on a footprint drawn on the floor. Footprints should be 2 inches apart from the center line.

3). Walk sideways. Begin the motor action with half steps. Perform the exercise rhythm (order): at one, shift the weight to the left foot; at two, place the right foot 12 inches to the right; at three, shift the weight to the right foot; at four, move the left foot over to the right foot. Repeat the exercise with half steps to the left.

Is it reasonable to schedule a full-day motor training?

Avoiding excessive fatigue is a principle during motor training, especially for stroke patients. The intensity and duration of motor training need to be determined according to the patient's tolerance.

Perceived exertion during the exercise may be learned by asking the patient. The magnitude of fatigue can also be known by observing the mental/physical state of the patient.

Two types of fatigue should be noticed, i.e., that occurs during the exercise and that still exists after the exercise. Excessive fatigue/exertion that occurs during the exercise may lead to the acute onset of cardiovascular/cerebrovascular diseases. Chronic fatigue hinders functional recovery and may also trigger a variety of diseases.

Note that some patients may feel mental fatigue before physical tiredness.

Do conventional exercises such as roller exercise benefit stroke patients?

Exercise using a roller, sanding board, and peg inserting board may be helpful when a ration force-exerting mode is applied. Especially, key components of reaching forward may be evoked during the training, such as shoulder protraction and elbow extension. A possible problem is that active shoulder flexion is not (or hardly) needed to complete a roller or sanding board exercise.

Thus, a recommended approach is to use roller and/or sanding board exercises as supplements to the reaching-forward training algorithm. Perform these exercises by using the same principles and try to initiate, enhance, or fine-grained control muscles for shoulder protraction, flexion, and elbow extension. The pegboard exercise may be arranged after roller and sanding board exercises since it needs better capacity.

Is reaching forward without arm flexion a meaningful exercise?

Normal arm and hand functions need both extension (reaching) and flexion control. In stroke patients, voluntary arm flexion often appears earlier and is stronger than arm extension. Additionally, arm extension control is much harder to be achieved in comparison with arm flexion. If a stroke patient can acquire a certain degree of reaching control, corresponding flexion control is easy to be trained. However, the reverse is not true.

As to the lower limb, most people have stronger leg extensors than flexors. However, standing and walking need very strong muscle control of leg extensors since lower limbs (mainly extensors) support the whole body weight during standing and walking. Thus, leg extensor training has a higher priority than flexors.

Are there any exercises to improve arm flexion control?

Fine-grained control exercise using the rational force-exerting mode can be performed to train arm flexors such as the brachialis and biceps brachii. The training involves a constant and relatively slow speed, proper alignment, and various types of muscle contractions (concentric, eccentric, and isometric). These exercises may improve the fine-tuning ability of the stronger muscles (dominant muscle groups in the arm and shoulder girdle).

The fine-grained control exercise may also be applied to other dominant muscle groups for a given motor action. The dominant muscle groups are usually antagonists or synergists to disturb proper alignment for a functional motor action, e.g., the latissimus dorsi for shoulder flexion, the elbow flexors for elbow extension, and the tibialis anterior for foot eversion during ankle dorsiflexion. However, note that enough forces generated by key muscles of a functional motor action play a crucial role in completing the activity, e.g., the serratus anterior, shoulder flexors, and elbow extensors in forward reaching. Thus, resources should be mainly assigned to improve the function of key muscles that complete key motor actions.

Is the proposed training protocol suitable for all stroke patients?

The algorithm for training walking ability may be used for almost all patients who cooperate well, but not all stroke patients have the potential to recover reaching control.

Long-lasting flaccidity usually indicates poor motor recovery in the upper and lower limbs. However, even though it is difficult to regain elbow, wrist, and hand control in some stroke patients, a functional shoulder protraction and other shoulder girdle movements, if regained, can protect the hemiplegic shoulder to some extent, and the required force-exerting mode during the training sessions can be transferred to other motor action training. In a rare condition when a patient regains good control of the shoulder and arm but not the hand, a universal cuff or similar devices may be applied to achieve some functions.

How to control spasticity?

Spasticity is considered as muscle tone increase due to hyperexcitability of the stretch reflex. It is featured by the velocity-dependent increase in the tonic stretch reflex. Clinically, spastic hemiplegia is used to indicate a constant state of muscle contraction on the hemiplegia side.

Both viscoelastic properties of muscle-tendon units and the neural control of muscles influence spasticity. Stretching can change viscoelastic properties and the shortening of the muscle and nearby soft tissues.

The neural component of spasticity originates from several reasons: 1) overflow effects due to weak agonists; 2) overactive muscle contractions of antagonists and synergists; and 3) abnormal spatial-temporal relation of muscle contractions.

Note that weakness of an agonist can be accompanied by the disturbance of the spatial-temporal relationship of contractions of the agonist: a hemiplegia patient initiates agonist contraction slower than a normal subject (i.e., the muscle force is not generated when the force should be); the duration of the contraction is too longer than a normal subject (i.e., the force gradually becomes larger when the generated force should be small, and the force still exists when it should disappear); at the same time, the absolute force of muscle contraction is lower than the normal state (e.g., the peak of the muscle force does not reach the normal level) [1, 6]. As the result, when a motor action is performed, the muscle force may be higher than the normal level in some periods (due to the slow increase of muscle force) and be lower in other periods (e.g., in the beginning, due to the slow initiation and insufficient strength of the muscle), which is how weakness and spasticity coexist in the same muscle. What also coexists is a slow response, i.e., a slow initiation of muscle contraction, a slow force-changing speed, and a slow termination of muscle contraction.

Taken together, a slow response, insufficient absolute contraction force (insufficient excitation), and insufficient inhibition are the three key reasons for hemiplegic muscle dysfunction. These deficits occur in the agonist, antagonist, and synergist of a motor action and lead to improper motor performance. Apparently, this is more complex than "selective" control.

CNS lesions after stroke destruct normal pathways so that motor commands cannot be accurately sent to target regions, which results in overflow effects (often accompanied by negative emotions). As a result, the decreased motor control capacity cannot cope with external constraints such as biomechanical and muscle biological factors and constraints from the environment.

Among these causes, the decreased force generation of the primary mover is crucial. There are many approaches to support body weight (of the arm, leg, or entire body) for improving motor performance in stroke patients. To improve their own capabilities of motor control, the force generation of the primary mover needs to be focused on: determine an important motor action first, and then determine the primary movers. Initiate voluntary muscle contraction, and then enhance the force generation. To avoid overflow, perform fine-grained control training. The enhancement and the fine-grained control training are often combined. This is the algorithm to cope with spasticity at the root.

May improper movement patterns appear during motor training?

The formation of the LTP and related neural plasticity needs repetition. During exercise, temporally appearing mild malalignment is therefore permitted if continuous improvement of the alignment can be achieved. This principle also applies to other elements of motor control, including whether motor actions are smooth, non-rigid, and coordinated. Thus, short-lived errors may occur during the motor training process if the general direction is correct. However, note that an improper force-exerting mode and resulted movement patterns may not be easily corrected once learned, especially for patients with more severe paralysis.

Also note that not all stroke patients have the potential to regain perfectly normal motor control, e.g., recover a normal gait. Under such a situation, certain components of functional motor actions have to be removed for the expectation. For example, perfect control of hip and knee flexors may not be acquired in some patients. However, this does not mean that long-lasting severe abnormal movement patterns should appear during training.

Why feel the movement when performing movement?

A rational force-exerting mode emphasizes "feeling" the movement. When initiating or enhancing muscle contractions, the proposed protocol uses specific sensations to guide the motor action. When exercising fine-grained control, the patient needs to "experience" the motor action.

The somatosensory system and motor system are tightly integrated on multiple levels. In the peripheral, sensory nerve fibers and motor nerve fibers enter the muscle spindle, where the sensitivity of the sensory nerve endings increases when intrafusal muscle fibers are contracting.

Muscle spindles are distributed in a wide area of the skeletal muscle and measure both the length and change of length of a muscle. They send afferent inputs to the brain as the origin of proprioception and play an important role in regulating muscle contractions by activating motor neurons via the stretch reflex to resist muscle stretch. There is also dynamic and static gamma motor innervation of muscle spindles [7]. In the CNS, thalamic neurons can relay sensory inputs (along the spinothalamic system) directly to M1 and CMA in addition to S1, S2, and other cortical areas [8]. This pathway provides a shortcut between sensory and motor systems [9]. Additionally, the reciprocal axonal projection between M1 and S1 allows S1 to directly drive some motor actions [10].

Sensorimotor integration has been introduced as a mechanism for many years. Here, an operable approach is proposed to improve motor control capacity.

References

[1] Rizzolatti G, Kalaska JF. Voluntary Movement: The Primary Motor Cortex. In: Kandel ER, Schwartz JH, Jessell TM, Siegelbaum SA, Hudspeth AJ eds. Principles of Neural Science. 2013. London. McGraw-Hill. 835-864.

[2] Kirkesola G. Neurac a new treatment method for long-term musculoskeletal pain. Fysioterapeuten. 2009; 76: 16-25.

[3] Janet HC, Roberta BS. A Motor Relearning Programme for Stroke. 1987. 2nd. Rockville, USA. Aspen Publishers.

[4] Davies PM. Steps to follow. 2000. 2nd. Wemding, Germany. Springer. 508.

[5] Wei P, Zhang Z, Lv Z, Jing B. Strong Functional Connectivity among Homotopic Brain Areas Is Vital for Motor Control in Unilateral Limb Movement. Front Hum Neurosci. 2017; 11: 366 - 10.3389/fnhum.2017.00366 [doi].

[6] Hoffman DS, Strick PL. Effects of a primary motor cortex lesion on step-tracking movements of the wrist. J Neurophysiol. 1995; 73: 891-5.

[7] Partanen JV, Vanhanen J, Liljander SK. Electromyography of the muscle spindle. Sci Rep. 2022; 12: 4220.

[8] Dum RP, Levinthal DJ, Strick PL. The spinothalamic system targets motor and sensory areas in the cerebral cortex of monkeys. J Neurosci. 2009; 29: 14223-35.

[9] Wei P, Bao R, Lv Z, Jing B. Weak but Critical Links between Primary Somatosensory Centers and Motor Cortex during Movement. Front Hum Neurosci. 2018; 12: 1 – 10.3389/fnhum.2018.00001 [doi].

[10] Matyas F, Sreenivasan V, Marbach F, et al. Motor Control by Sensory Cortex. Science; 2010; 330: 1240-1243.

Screening cognitive impairment

Key points

- This chapter introduces a brief screening instrument for assessing cognitive function after stroke and other neurological diseases.
- This tool may also be used as a screening scale for detecting mild cognitive dysfunction (MCI or cognitive decline milder than MCI).
- In this tool, a graded-difficulty memory assessment is adopted in the item "Word Recall."

Cognitive function plays an important role in motor rehabilitation for stroke patients. It will be convenient to quickly assessing cognitive function of stroke patients before determining/adjusting therapeutic programs.

Additionally, cognitive impairment and dementia are commonly caused by mixed pathologies including Alzheimer's disease and cerebral vascular diseases. The brain pathologies may exist several decades before onset of dementia. Early detection of mild cognition decline can therefore contribute to better prevention of all-cause cognitive impairment and relieve risks of vascular dementia and AD later in life. For stroke patients, a tool for screening cognitive impairment can also measure changes in cognitive function during rehabilitation.

In this chapter, some components in a cognition assessment instrument are introduced, and a screening tool is designed to quickly and sensitively detect mild cognition dysfunction.

Cognitive dysfunction has adverse effects on motor rehabilitation after stroke

Cognitive dysfunction often occurs in stroke patients and has a negative impact on motor rehabilitation [1]. Decline of cognitive function is common in stroke patients. Stroke may cause mild cognitive impairment (MCI) and dementia [2]. Even for patients 3 months after minor strokes, motor performance is found to be associated with cognitive function [3]. After onset of stroke, better motor recovery in the acute and subacute phases is followed by better cognitive status [4]. Compared with motor training alone, cognitive training combined with motor rehabilitation programs can achieve better cognitive and motor function [5].

Brain lesions caused by stroke interfere with the functional interaction between brain regions, and thus influence both motor performance and cognitive function. Stroke patients need to regain motor skills, muscular strength and endurance. The motor learning process involves multiple cognitive functions including memory, planning, attention, and execution. The higher brain functions rely upon the ability to integrate information across many brain regions. These brain regions form several modules (groups) performing different functions with some degree of independence. During different states when performing a cognitive task, the original modular structure may be enhanced [6]. For instance, posture control during turning around and sitting down requires more cognitive resources and stroke patients with cognitive deficits need more time to perform these movements, thereby presenting impaired balance and higher fall risk [7]. Additionally, it is challenging for patients with mild stroke to rapidly respond to changing conditions during complex reaching tasks. Such deficit is possibly related to cognitive deficits and limitations in the regulation of tonic stretch reflex. The problem needs be considered during rehabilitation and the integration of the hemiplegic arm into activities of daily living should be encouraged [8].

Cognitive impairment does not affect only functions of stroke patients. A study with 1996 subjects aged ≥55 years find that each 5-point decrease in the mini mental state examination (MMSE) score was associated with a 34% increased risk of all-cause mortality and a 56% increased risk of cardiovascular disease mortality[9]. Even in older adults without manifested dementia, subjects with low cognitive test scores had approximately 60% increased mortality compared with those with higher test scores. Cognitive impairment in the absence of manifest dementia is an important independent predictor of mortality, suggesting that it is crucial to learn cognitive status in older adults is for health care and treatment decisions [10].

A tool for rapid assessing cognitive function in stroke patients is needed

A simple, easily performed tool is needed to measure cognitive function in stroke patients. With this instrument, one can quickly know the cognitive level of a stroke patient. A short scale will not be a burden for patients and can be retested easily. Additionally, a scale with good sensitivity may detect changes in cognitive function in a short period.

There are two types of instruments to measure cognitive function. One is based on the performance of patients/subjects such as the mini mental state examination (MMSE) and the Montreal Cognitive Assessment (MoCA), and the other is the informant-based measure such as AD8. The performance-based scales are often unable to detect changes in cognitive function between the current state and previous levels of a subject. Some performance-based measures are also insensitive to quantify subtle changes in individuals with high cognitive function in the early stages of dementia. As an informant-based instrument, AD8 is sensitive in detecting early cognitive decline, whereas a good informant (living together with the patients, especially spouses) may not be readily available [11].

For stroke patients, informant-based measures are usually not used to quantify cognitive function since (1) for patients with mild cognitive impairments, an informant is often unable to provide useful information and may overestimate the cognitive level of the patient, and (2) for patients with severe cognitive dysfunction, the cognition decline can be easily determined by medical professionals.

Performance-based scales such as MMSE and MoCA are often used to assess cognitive function in stroke patients. The highest possible score is 30 points for each instrument. Both tests assess executive function, memory, language, attention, computation, and orientation. Compared with MMSE, MoCA has more complex items for testing language and attention and evaluates more cognitive domains including visuoconstructional skills, conceptual thinking, and concentration.

A meta-analysis finds that MMSE is not as sensitive as MoCA for assessing mild cognitive impairment (MCI) among elderly people $\geqslant$ 60 years. The cut-off point of MoCA is 24/25 (sensitivity, 80.48%; specificity, 81.19%), whereas the best cut-off of MMSE is 27/28 (sensitivity, 66.34%; specificity, 72.94%) [12]. The approximation between the cut-off value 27/28 and the full score 30 indicates that MMSE has a ceiling effect. In other words, MMSE cannot differentiate individuals with relatively high cognition levels because the items of MMSE lack enough challenges. The lower cut-off point of MoCA stems from more cognitive domains and higher difficulty of items than MMSE.

Normal young people often take less than 10 minutes to complete the MoCA test. However, stroke patients with cognitive impairments may need a much longer time to complete the MoCA test, which makes the test unsuitable to be used as a brief instrument for examining stroke patients with cognitive states worse than MCI.

Components of cognitive function assessment

A good instrument to rapidly assess cognitive function for stroke patients should meet several requirements:

(1) The content of the scale is brief, and the test can be completed within several minutes.
(2) The scale can be easily performed, e.g., as a pencil-paper test.
(3) The scale assesses several key components of cognitive function.
(4) The scale can provide enough level of challenge to avoid the ceiling effect.

(5) Individuals with poor cognitive function may get a certain score to avoid the floor effect.
(6) Items of the scale can acquire as much information as possible from the patients.
(7) The scale is sensitive to detect changes after treatment.
(8) The scale has a standardized operating interface, a standardized guideline, and scoring rules.
(9) The scale contents can be applied with different languages with a consistent meaning.

It is common to design a performance-based instrument with a "building-blocks" approach using classic cognitive tests. For example, MMSE contains a 3-word recall, time and place orientation, 3-object naming, sentence repetition, following verbal and written commands, write a sentence, subtraction (serial 7s), and copying intersecting pentagons [13]. These items come from the mentor of the author and some textbooks [14].

Consistency is important when performing a test because it is hard to compare results from inconsistent operations. For instance, at present, there are various versions of MMSE. The contents of the MMSE test from different sources may vary to some extent, e.g., the shapes of the two intersecting pentagons are often different from that of the original version. Besides a pencil and paper, performing MMSE also needs a card with "CLOSE YOUR EYES" written on it, two objects for naming, and possibly an additional paper for testing the 3-stage command "Take a paper in your right hand, fold it in half, and put it on the floor". However, the examiner may perform these contents in different ways, e.g., using an oral command but not a card showing "Close your eyes". Such inconsistency among operations leads to difficulties when comparing results from different centres and examiners.

To prevent inconsistency among different operators, a standardized layout of the test and an administration/scoring instruction are needed (e.g., as provided by MoCA).

Several components of MoCA present higher challenge levels than those in MMSE. MoCA used a 5-word recall rather than a 3-word memory test. Additionally, MoCA supplemented several new components including the copy of cube test, trail making test, random letter test, and clock drawing test.

The copy of cube test is a classic cognitive test and may be more difficult than copying intersecting pentagons (**Figure 1**). The copy of cube test requires the subject to draw an identical cube including parallel lines and right angles [15], whereas copying intersecting pentagons only requires presenting all 10 angles with 2 angle intersecting [13]. The supplemented tests in MoCA contribute to its increased sensitivity [12, 16] than MMSE.

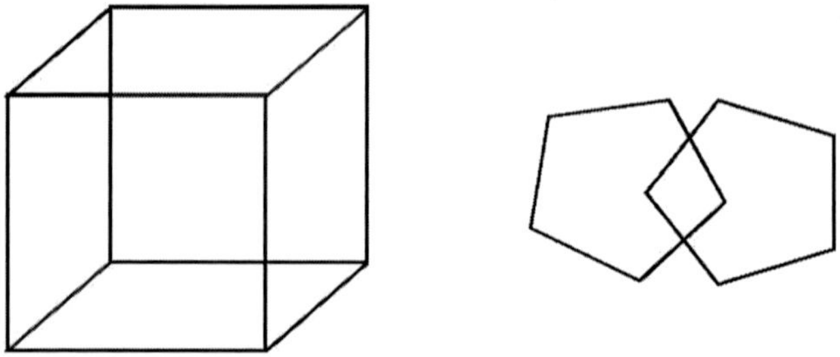

Figure 1. Cube and intersecting pentagons.

A copying/drawing test has several advantages. To complete a trail-making test, clock drawing test, or copying a graph (cube or pentagons) similar to a Bender-Gestalt figure, the subject needs to use visuoconstructional skills and executive functions. Visuospatial function impairments cause difficulties in spatial orientation during movements, problems in spatial coordination, perception of the relative size of objects, and spatial distances and positions, and thus disturb sensorimotor interaction [17]. Additionally, a drawing test such as the Bender-Gestalt test or House-Tree-Person test may reveal some aspects of personality and mood [18, 19]. Therefore, the behavior of the subject during the test together with the performance of the drawing may reveal the comprehensive state of a subject.

Trail making test

The trail-making test comprises two components, Part A and Part B. In Part A, the subject is asked to connect numbers with lines in a numerical sequence (i.e., 1–2–3–…); Part B requires the subject to draw lines to connect numbers and letters in an alternating numeric and alphabetic sequence (i.e., 1–A–2–B–3–C–…). Part A is a visuomotor sequence tracking task, and the Part B additionally examines the flexibility of set-switching between numbers and letters. Lesions in a number of brain regions including the left rostral anterior cingulate, prefrontal cortex, and insula lead to poor performance of Part B, indicating the engagement of multiple brain areas to the task [20]. Note that variance in time to completing Part B is uniquely impacted by visuomotor scanning, whereas working memory and executive functioning contributes to the error score of Part B [21].

Average durations to completing the test Part B for normal aging, MCI, and dementia people in the age of 70s are 81.5±36.1 seconds, 136±78 seconds, and 190±81.6 seconds; average errors (errors are incorrect lines reaching its target) for the normal aging, mild cognitive impairment, and dementia people are 0.45±0.85, 1.05±1.22, and 1.39 ±1.31. The performance error rate of Part B can differentiate normal aging from MCI or AD but not MCI from AD, whereas the completion time can differentiate normal aging, MCI, and AD (normal aging <MCI<AD all $p<0.001$). The sensitivity for MCI vs. normal aging is 43% but the specificity can reach 91.1% [22]. In short, the completion time of Part B can be used to differentiate normal elderly people from MCI but the sensitivity (i.e., the proportion of the disordered group correctly identified by the test) is low. Similarly, a low sensitivity for MCI vs. normal aging was also revealed in another study where the area under the ROC curve is only 0.70 (95% CI = 0.67–0.73) for Part B [23]. The low sensitivity of Part B for MCI vs. normal aging suggests that increasing the challenge level of the test may be considered.

Cultural context results in bias in performance which is a challenge for cognitive tests currently used in healthcare and research settings [24]. Due to culture/language factors, in some countries the letters have to be changed (e.g., to Chinese or Japanese characters). Other forms of sets rather than letters may also be needed for subjects with low education levels. Here, we recommend a trail- making test without letters and numbers and therefore can be easily applied to subjects using all languages (**Figure 2**).

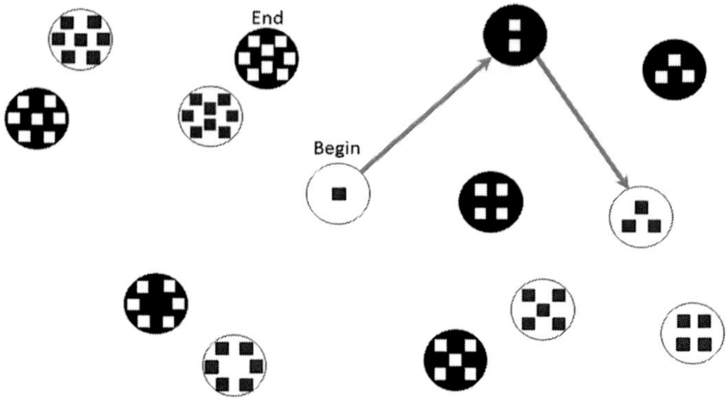

Figure 2. Recommended trail-making test.

Instruction: Draw a line in ascending order, as the two arrows show. Begin here (pointing to the word "Begin"). End here (pointing to the word "End").

Copy of cube test

The copy of cube test is part of the Short Test of Mental Status (STMS) [25]. Compared with MMSE, the STMS was better for detecting MCI and was more sensitive in detecting cognitive deficits in individuals who had normal cognition at baseline but later developed MCI or AD [26].

Several representative results of the test are shown in **Figure 3**, including two different types of rectangular prism, right rectangular prism (1, 2, and 3 in **Figure 3**) and non-right rectangular prism (4 in **Figure 3**). The shapes of 3 and 4 are quite different from a cube and thus are abnormal results although result 3 is a right rectangular prism. A detailed scoring criterion of the copy of cube test is introduced in [15]. Here, simple instruction and scoring criteria are presented.

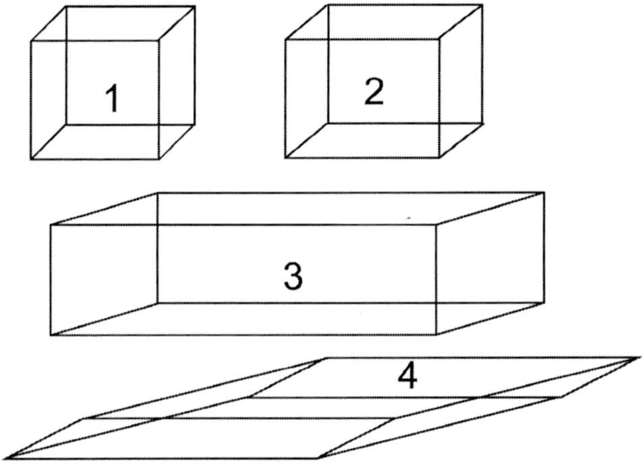

Figure 3. Copy of cube test.

1. Correct; 2. Acceptable; 3 and 4, abnormal.

Instruction: Copy the drawing as exactly as you can. Scoring criteria: No missing lines or added lines; all angles should be right (90 degrees); the shape is close to the template.

Calculation

A calculation test is often included in a screening instrument for detecting cognitive impairment. The "Serial 7s" is a commonly-used calculation test.

To complete the test, the subject is instructed to subtract 7 from 100 and stop after 5 answers. The test examines attention and calculation. However, some subjects may not understand the requirement and stop after one or two operations. Additionally, subtraction is only one form of calculation and may not be able to sensitively detect cognitive decline in the calculation.

Orientation

Orientation is a traditionally defined cognitive domain and often included in screening tests such as MMSE, MoCA, and STMS. The Clinical Dementia Rating (CDR) examines 6 domains of cognitive and functional performance through interviewing the patient and an informant, i.e., memory, orientation, judgment & problem solving, community affairs, home & hobbies, and personal care. In amnestic MCI individuals, the CDR orientation score predicts AD dementia progression more accurately than either the logistic regression analyses model with either MMSE or CDR sum scores [27].

The MMSE orientation section contains five spatial orientation and five temporal orientation items. In the linear multiple regression analyses in subjects with MCI and AD, the orientation score was predicted by worse performance on immediate and delayed recall, by decreased entorhinal cortex thickness, hippocampal volume, and inferior temporal cortex thickness, and by glucose hypometabolism in middle-inferior temporal cortex and hippocampus. After 4 years of follow-up, disoriented MCI subjects (>8 scores) presented almost 1.5 times the risk of AD conversion in comparison with oriented subjects (≤8 scores). Temporal disorientation

(18%) but not spatial disorientation (9%) accounted for most of the explained variance [28]. These results suggest that the orientation score in MCI subjects is a risk factor for progression to AD, especially the temporal part. In a study that enrolled 505 elderly subjects (mean age 85 years), temporal orientation was also found to be the only domain significantly associated with MMSE decline over time [29]. Another study find that two temporal orientation items, date and day of week, were inversely associated with AD progression in MCI subjects whereas other temporal orientation items (year, month, and season), as well as all five spatial orientation items, cannot provide information on prediction [30].

Quick-Cog test for screening cognitive function

The Quick-Cog Basic test is a screening instrument for detecting mild cognitive dysfunction in adults. It can be used as a screening tool to assess cognitive function in the community or as a bedside screening tool for stroke patients.

Similar to other cognitive tests, the Quick-Cog Basic test is a package containing several components, including two types of word recall tests, a clock drawing test, and a trail-making test.

A young adult with the risk of dementia may present reduced cognitive performance 40 years before the typical onset of AD [31]. Thus, it is necessary to develop tools for quickly and *sensitively* detecting cognitive decline in adults including elderly and younger people. The memory test in the Quick-Cog test aims to increase the challenge level of immediate/delayed recall. Similarly, a trail-making test is designed to provide increased difficulty by using *concise* instruction; the instruction does not tell a subject to alternately connect two different types of targets with lines, and the subject must find the correct pattern by himself (herself).

To avoid across-cultural differences, seven commonly-used words are selected in the memory test and no letters and numbers are used in the trail-making test.

A sensitive screening tool for detecting mild cognitive dysfunction in adults is *urgently* needed. Thus, enhancing sensitivity is the top priority when designing the Quick-Cog test. The Quick-Cog test is designed for screening instruments for *quickly* and *sensitively* detecting mild cognitive dysfunction in adults including elderly and younger people. Here, mild cognitive dysfunction means a deficit possibly even milder than MCI.

MCI is not the beginning of AD. Cognitive function such as verbal learning and memory performance may be slightly impaired forty years (at 18 years old) before the typical onset of AD [31]; the impairment is very mild and cannot be classified as MCI during that period. Thus, it is necessary to detect slightly cognitive decline in a very early stage and active interventions can be timely initiated.

As a simple screening tool, the Quick-Cog Basic test can be completed in a shorter duration than MMSE and MoCA. The Quick-Cog Basic test contains a challenging memory test even for young adults. Additionally, the trail-making test in the Quick-Cog Basic test is more difficult than its usual form. These items increase the test difficulty and therefore mild cognitive deficits may be detected. Such design (to increase sensitivity) stems from heavy burdens from dementia including AD and vascular dementia.

Dementia caused by AD, vascular dementia, and other reasons inflicts a heavy burden on society. Over 46 million people suffered from dementia worldwide in 2015. By 2050, the number is estimated to increase to 131.5 million [32]. Dementia is a very costly disease since there is no effective therapy and patients need expensive care for years. AD is the major cause of dementia accounting for over 50% of cases. Most developed drugs for AD were found to be ineffective and many related clinical trials were terminated. The burden of the US health care system from Alzheimer's and other dementias may reach 1 trillion US dollars each year at 2050 and result in a meltdown in the health-care system [33]. Between 2015 and 2050, the prevalence of dementia in high-income countries will increase by 116%, whereas the prevalence in upper-middle-income countries will increase by 227%, in lower-middle-income countries by 223%, and in low-income countries by 264% [32]. That means a tougher situation in less developed countries. The costs are projected to exceed those of all other chronic diseases. The rapidly rising tide of the incurable, costly diseases leads to a statement "We're faced with a tsunami and we're trying to deal with it with a bucket" [33].

Mixed pathologies in dementia patients have been commonly detected. AD may coexist with vascular dementia and other types of dementia including Lewy body dementia and hyperphosphorylated transactive response DNA-binding protein 43 (TDP-43) proteinopathy [34]. It is one of the reasons that a screening tool may be used for community-dwelling people and patients such as those with stroke.

Early detection of dementia is important because it is a good time window to receipt of health care services to delay and slow progression of related pathological changes [35]. Firstly, cognitive training such as video games can be used to optimize brain function and delay cognitive deficits in the aging population. Three-dimensional video game training can enhance cognitive function in 60-85 years older adults, and the effects persist for 6 months [36]. In 2,832 persons with mean age of 73.6 years, specific types of cognitive training (reasoning and speed, but not memory, training) can result in fewer declines in self-reported instrumental activities of daily living (IADL) in comparison with the control group for 10 years [37]. Secondly, the increase in educational attainment and healthy lifestyle contribute to a lower risk for dementia. When comparing data from a nationally representative, population-based longitudinal survey of individuals in the United States from 2000 (10, 546 subjects) and 2012 (10, 511 subjects), average years of education were found to increase from 11.8 years to 12.7 years between 2000 and 2012, whereas dementia prevalence among people 65 years or older decreased from 11.6% in 2000 to 8.8% in 2012 [38]. A UK study including 196 383 subjects aged ⩾60 years finds that among older adults without cognitive impairment or dementia, the disapproving lifestyle and high genetic risk are both significantly associated with a higher risk of dementia. Notably, a healthy lifestyle including no current smoking, regular physical activity, healthy diet, and moderate alcohol consumption, is associated with lower dementia risk among participants with high genetic risk [39].

Hence, increasing the coverage of timely dementia diagnosis is a priority for most national and regional policies and plans [35]. Although therapies and drugs that block or reverse the pathological progression of dementia are still lacking, the incidence rate of dementia in the United States and several developed countries in Europe has declined by 13% per decade over the past 25 years, consistently across 7 population-based cohort studies [40]. This finding may partially attribute to better education and healthcare support in these countries.

Interventions for reducing modifiable risk factors can lead to better control of the worldwide prevalence of dementia. Dementia primarily occurs in late life. Thus, delaying the onset by targeting modifiable risk factors should have a major impact on dementia prevalence. Using multi-domain interventions to correct dementia risk factors such as physical inactivity, unhealthy diet, cognitive inactivity, depression, anxiety, overweight/obesity, excess alcohol consumption, smoking, and chronic health conditions, a 2-year delay may reduce AD prevalence by up to 20%, and postponing the onset by 5 years may reduce AD prevalence in half [41].

However, dementia is currently under-detected, underdiagnosed, under-treated, and under-managed. Only 40-50% of dementia patients have received a diagnosis even in most high-income countries. In low- and middle-income countries, the diagnostic coverage may be less than 5-10% in most situations [35].

Pathogenesis of Alzheimer's disease is a continuous progression process. The brain pathological changes of AD occur several decades before dementia and MCI. A young adult with the risk of dementia may present reduced cognitive performance 40 years before the typical onset of Alzheimer's disease [31].

Approaches for screening dementia in the community

For achieving detection of dementia at the earliest stages, various approaches have been being developed. One type of approaches uses imaging, CSF, plasma, and retinal biomarkers for diagnosis, stratification, and determining progression of dementia, e.g., to identify and validate biomarkers for the small vessel diseases of the brain that produce vascular contributions to cognitive impairment and dementia (VCID) [42-44]. The other type of approach evaluates cognitive function of the subject. There are two types of instruments to measure cognitive function. One is based on the performance of patients/subjects such as MMSE and MoCA, and the other is the informant-based measure such as AD8.

The Quick-Cog test is a performance-based test. For stroke patients, such a tool can also measure changes in cognitive function during rehabilitation.

Contents of the Quick-Cog Basic test and examples of results from stroke patients

Figure 4 shows results of the Quick-Cog Basic test from a male patient suffering from a cerebral haemorrhage in the left parietal lobe (see the CT scan) two weeks after onset, demonstrating mild hemiplegia on the right side. The duration to complete the clock drawing was 61 seconds, and the instructions were repeated twice. He successfully remembered one word in the 3-word immediate recall, three words in the 5-word immediate recall, and three words in the 5-word immediate recall. He failed to remember any words in the delayed recall test but only repeated "clock, hour hand, minute hand" instructed during the former part (the clock-drawing test).

The immediate recall test, especially the 7-word, can mimic a digit span test to some extent and reflect attention in addition to memory.

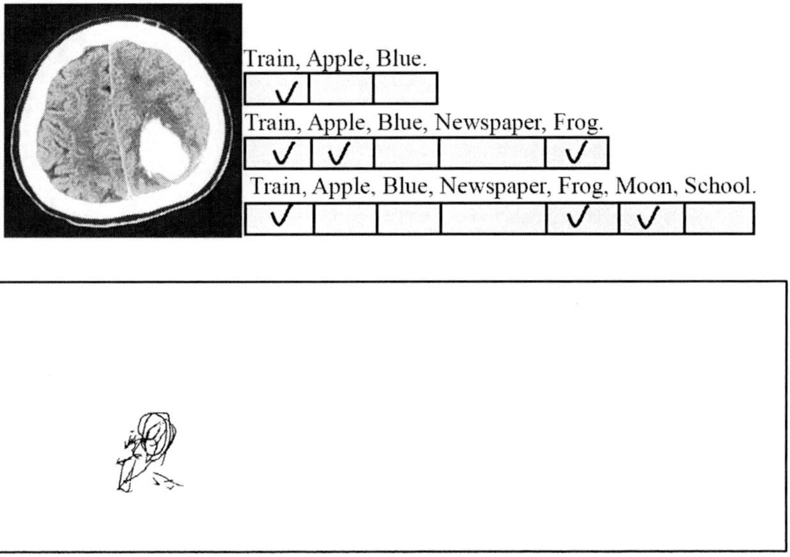

Figure 4 Results of the Quick-Cog Basic test from a young stroke patient.

Figure 5 shows results from an 84-years old patient suffering from cerebral infarction and mild hemiplegia on the right side. From the top to bottom, results of immediate recall, the clock-drawing test, and delayed recall are presented. The patient presented a good immediate recall and attention, whereas he could only remember one word in the delayed recall. Note that the only word remembered during the delayed recall is what was forgotten during the 7-word immediate recall. This reflected an internal retrieving process of the forgotten word, and such a process inhibited retrieving other words.

Note that the Quick-Cog test aims to examine cognitive function. Stroke patients should use the non-hemiplegic to complete the clock drawing, whereas community-dwelling subjects without hemiplegia routinely use the dominant to complete this test. The smoothness of lines drawn by non-dominant hands reflects motor impairments rather than cognitive dysfunction.

Train, Apple, Blue.

√	√	√

Train, Apple, Blue, Newspaper, Frog.

√	√	√	√	√

Train, Apple, Blue, Newspaper, Frog, Moon, School.

√	√		√	√	√	√

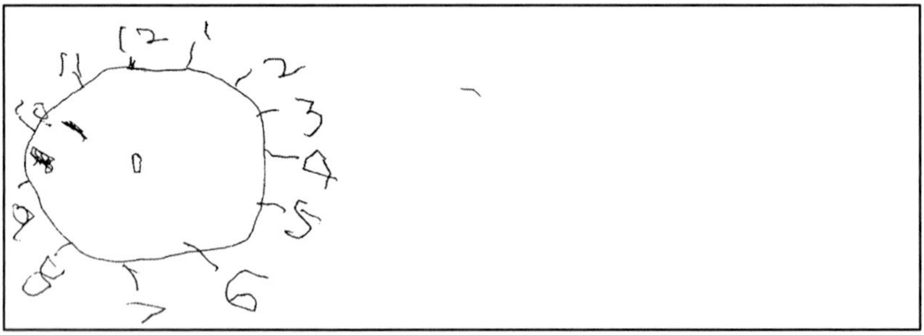

Train, Apple, Blue, Newspaper, Frog, Moon, School.

		√				

Figure 5 Results of the Quick-Cog Basic test from an old patient.

In the results of the clock-drawing test, the contour of the circle may be classified as graphical difficulties possibly indicating disruption of frontostriatal circuits to coordinate fine motor control and planning [45]. However, whether the circle is closed or drawn perfectly may not be a factor reflecting cognitive function but often indicate the compliance of the subject based on our experience. An active, impatient subject with good cognitive function may draw a circle rapidly with an apparently distorted circle. Therefore, the Quick-Cog test does not score the shape of the circle.

The total score of the Quick-Cog Basic test may not be used to judge whether a subject is normal. For a normal adult, recalling five words is the lower limit for immediate recall and delayed recall. In the community screening, a subject should get a full score and complete the clock-drawing test or the modified trail-making test within one minute. Otherwise, a more detailed cognitive test should be performed. In a US study performed in the community-dwelling people, the digital clock drawing test was completed during 39.26±16.91 seconds by 24 young adults aged 40.04±6.00 years and during 35.91±12.70 seconds for by 28 older adults aged 66.04±4.10 years [46]. Similarly, 20 healthy subjects aged 66.9±9.4 years completed the clock drawing during 49.2284±10.3581 seconds in a German study [47]. For subjects with motor dysfunction or using non-dominant hands, the time limit needs to be studied. The completion time for the trail-making time increases with growing age and fewer years of education [48], and the normal value for the different groups needs to be determined.

Appendix: Quick-Cog Basicv2.1 and 2.2

Quick-Cog Basic v2.1 is now used for screening cognitive function of stroke patients, and Quick-Cog Basic v2.2 for community screening, especially for young adults. A 3-word recall test and a clock drawing test cannot provide enough challenges to young people. Hence, a longer list of words, a clock drawing, and a modified trail-making test are combined.

A longer list of words is used to increase sensitivity, and a modified trail-making test is used because the specificity of the test for MCI vs. normal aging can reach 91.1% [22].

Quick-Cog Basic v2.1

Name:

Sex: Age: Education:

1. Immediate Recall

Remember the three words (one per second): Train, Apple, Blue.
Tell me these words: [ ] [ ] [ ]

Remember the five words (one per second): Train, Apple, Blue, Newspaper, Frog.
Tell me these words: [ ] [ ] [ ] [ ] [ ]

Remember the seven words (one per second): Train, Apple, Blue, Newspaper, Frog, Moon, School.
Tell me these words: [ ] [ ] [ ] [ ] [ ] [ ] [ ]

2. Clock Drawing

(Fold the paper along the lines.) Draw a round clock face. Put all the numbers in the correct positions. Place clock hands at "10 minutes after 11". (The maximum allowable time is 3 minutes.)

How many times the Instruction is said: _____

How long it takes to complete the clock drawing: _____ seconds.

All 12 correct numbers are shown. [ ]

All the numbers are placed in the correct positions. [ ]

Clock hands are placed at "10 minutes after 11". [ ]

3. Delayed Recall

I asked you to remember some words. Tell me these words:
Train, Apple, Blue, Newspaper, Frog, Moon, School.

[ ] [ ] [ ] [ ] [ ] [ ] [ ]

Total score ____/10

Examiner:________ Date: ___________

Quick-Cog Basic v2.2

Name:

Sex: Age: Education:

1. Immediate Recall

Remember the three words (one per second): Train, Apple, Blue.
Tell me these words:

Remember the five words (one per second): Train, Apple, Blue, Newspaper, Frog.
Tell me these words:

Remember the seven words (one per second): Train, Apple, Blue, Newspaper, Frog, Moon, School.
Tell me these words:

2. Timed Clock Drawing

Draw a round clock face. Put all the numbers in the correct positions. Place clock hands at "10 minutes after 11".
(The maximum allowable time is 3 minutes.)

3. Timed Trail Making

White circles contain increasing numbers of squares, so do black circles. The two arrows link three circles. Draw a line in the same pattern. Begin here (pointing to the word "Begin"). End here (pointing to the word "End"). (2 minutes.)

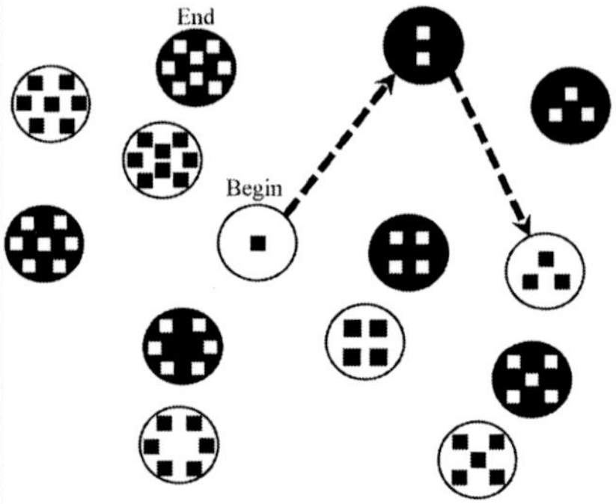

How long to complete the task: _____ seconds.

All 12 correct numbers are shown.

All numbers in the correct positions.

Clock hands placed at "10 after 11".

How long to complete the task: _____ seconds.

The correct connections are shown.

Correct and no self-corrections.

4. Delayed Recall

I asked you to remember some words. Tell me these words:

Train, Apple, Blue, Newspaper, Frog, Moon, School.

Total score ____/12

Examiner:________ Date: ___________

Instructions for Administration and Scoring

The Quick-Cog Basic v2.1 and v2.2 are screening instruments for detecting mild cognitive dysfunction. Print the Quick-Cog Basic on an A4 paper and perform the test based on the following instructions.

1. Immediate Recall

Read the words in blue. Firstly, say: "Remember the three words", and say: "Train, Apple, Blue" at a rate of approximately one second for each of the three words. After that, tell the subject: "Tell me these words". As shown by the words in red, check the allocated box for each word correctly repeated by the subject. Read the next sentence in blue when the subject has recalled all three words or indicates that he/she cannot recall all words.

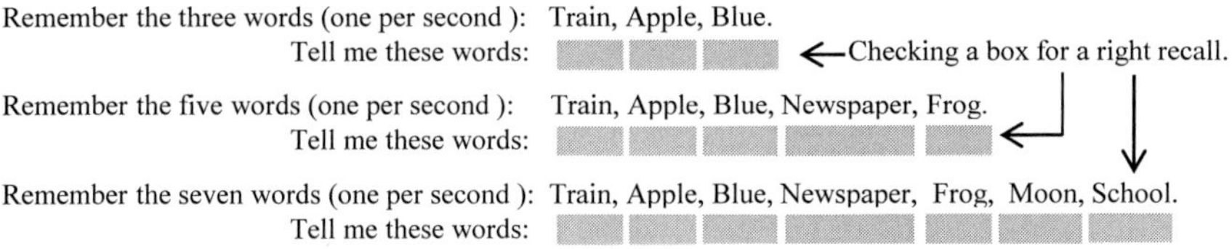

The instructions are read only once.

This part examines immediate memory over a period of seconds [49]. Similar to a digit span test, listening and repeating the three lists of words may also measure attention.

Scoring: No points for this part.

2. Timed Clock Drawing

Fold the paper along the lines. Present only the blank part of the paper to the subject.

Instruct the subject: "Draw a round clock face. Put all the numbers in the correct positions. Place clock hands at 10 minutes after 11." Start timing after this instruction.

The maximum allowable time is 3 minutes. Move to the next part if the drawing is not completed in 3 minutes.

Scoring: One point is assigned for each of the following responses:

- All 12 correct numbers are shown.
- All the numbers are placed in the correct positions.
- Clock hands are placed at "10 minutes after 11".

3. Timed Trail Making

Present only the part of the trail-making test to the subject.

Instruct the subject: "The two arrows link three circles. Draw a line in the same pattern. Begin here [pointing to the word (Begin)]. End here [pointing to the word (End)]." Start timing after this instruction.

The maximum allowable time is 2 minutes. Move to the next part if the drawing is not completed in 2 minutes.

Scoring: One point is assigned for each of the following responses:

- The correct connections are shown.
- No self-corrections (one point is given only if all connections are correct).

4. Delayed Recall

Instruct the subject: "I asked you to remember some words. Tell me these words."

Do not present any cues. Check the allocated box for each word correctly recalled by the subject.

Scoring: One point is assigned for each word recalled correctly.

Interpreting the score of the Quick-Cog Basic

The scores of items 2 and 4 are added together for Quick-Cog Basic v2.1, and the scores of items 2, 3, and 4 are added together for Quick-Cog Basic v2.2. Note that the weight of the memory test in the sum score is superior to other tests.

In addition to the score, the speed to complete a test (the Clock Drawing or the Trail Making) is also a useful parameter.

A young adult with the risk of dementia may present reduced cognitive performance 40 years before the typical onset of Alzheimer's disease. Thus, it is necessary to develop tools for quickly and *sensitively* detecting cognitive decline in adults including elderly and younger people. The memory test in the Quick-Cog Basic aims to increase the challenge level of immediate/delayed recall. Similarly, the Trail Making test is designed to provide increased difficulty by using a concise guide.

To avoid across-cultural differences, seven common words are used in the memory test and no letters and numbers are used in the trail-making test.

References

[1] Aprile I, Guardati G, Cipollini V, et al. Influence of Cognitive Impairment on the Recovery of Subjects with Subacute Stroke Undergoing Upper Limb Robotic Rehabilitation. Brain Sci. 2021. 11(5).

[2] Allan HR, Brown RH. Adams and Victor's Principles of Neurology. 2005. 8th ed. New York. McGraw-Hill. 380-382.

[3] Einstad MS, Saltvedt I, Lydersen S, et al. Associations between post-stroke motor and cognitive function: a cross-sectional study. BMC Geriatr. 2021. 21(1): 103.

[4] French MA, Cohen ML, Pohlig RT, Reisman DS. Fluid Cognitive Abilities Are Important for Learning and Retention of a New, Explicitly Learned Walking Pattern in Individuals After Stroke. Neurorehabil Neural Repair. 2021: 15459683211001025.

[5] Eschweiler M, Bohr L, Kessler J, Fink GR, Kalbe E, Onur OA. Combined cognitive and motor training improves the outcome in the early phase after stroke and prevents a decline of executive functions: A pilot study. NeuroRehabilitation. 2021. 48(1): 97-108.

[6] Shine JM, Bissett PG, Bell PT, et al. The Dynamics of Functional Brain Networks: Integrated Network States during Cognitive Task Performance. Neuron. 2016. 92(2): 544-554.

[7] Yu HX, Wang ZX, Liu CB, Dai P, Lan Y, Xu GQ. Effect of Cognitive Function on Balance and Posture Control after Stroke. Neural Plast. 2021. 2021: 6636999.

[8] Hasanbarani F, Batalla M, Feldman AG, Levin MF. Mild Stroke Affects Pointing Movements Made in Different Frames of Reference. Neurorehabil Neural Repair. 2021. 35(3): 207-219.

[9] An J, Li H, Tang Z, et al. Cognitive Impairment and Risk of All-Cause and Cardiovascular Disease Mortality Over 20-Year Follow-up: Results From the BLSA. J Am Heart Assoc. 2018. 7(15): e008252.

[10] Perna L, Wahl HW, Mons U, Saum KU, Holleczek B, Brenner H. Cognitive impairment, all-cause and cause-specific mortality among non-demented older adults. Age Ageing. 2015. 44(3): 445-51.

[11] Galvin JE, Roe CM, Powlishta KK, et al. The AD8: a brief informant interview to detect dementia. Neurology. 2005. 65(4): 559-64.

[12] Ciesielska N, Sokołowski R, Mazur E, Podhorecka M, Polak-Szabela A, Kędziora-Kornatowska K. Is the Montreal Cognitive Assessment (MoCA) test better suited than the Mini-Mental State Examination (MMSE) in mild cognitive impairment (MCI) detection among people aged over 60? Meta-analysis. Psychiatr Pol. 2016. 50(5): 1039-1052.

[13] Folstein MF, Folstein SE, McHugh PR. "Mini-mental state". A practical method for grading the cognitive state of patients for the clinician. J Psychiatr Res. 1975. 12(3): 189-98.

[14] Folstein M. Mini-mental and son. Int J Geriatr Psychiatry. 1998. 13(5): 290-4.

[15] Fountoulakis KN, Siamouli M, Magiria S, et al. A standardized scoring method for the copy of cube test, developed to be suitable

for use in psychiatric populations. Ann Gen Psychiatry. 2011. 10(1): 19.

[16] Ghafar M, Miptah HN, O'Caoimh R. Cognitive screening instruments to identify vascular cognitive impairment: A systematic review. Int J Geriatr Psychiatry. 2019. 34(8): 1114-1127.

[17] Mukundan CR. Computerized Cognitive Retraining Programs for Patients Afflicted with Traumatic Brain Injury and Other Brain Disorders. 2013. Oxford.

[18] Brannigan GG, Decker SL. The Bender-Gestalt II. Am J Orthopsychiatry. 2006. 76(1): 10-2.

[19] Sheng L, Yang G, Pan Q, Xia C, Zhao L. Synthetic House-Tree-Person Drawing Test: A New Method for Screening Anxiety in Cancer Patients. J Oncol. 2019. 2019: 5062394.

[20] Varjacic A, Mantini D, Demeyere N, Gillebert CR. Neural signatures of Trail Making Test performance: Evidence from lesion-mapping and neuroimaging studies. Neuropsychologia. 2018. 115: 78-87.

[21] Mahurin RK, Velligan DI, Hazleton B, Mark Davis J, Eckert S, Miller AL. Trail making test errors and executive function in schizophrenia and depression. Clin Neuropsychol. 2006. 20(2): 271-88.

[22] Ashendorf L, Jefferson AL, O'Connor MK, Chaisson C, Green RC, Stern RA. Trail Making Test errors in normal aging, mild cognitive impairment, and dementia. Arch Clin Neuropsychol. 2008. 23(2): 129-37.

[23] Wei M, Shi J, Li T, et al. Diagnostic Accuracy of the Chinese Version of the Trail-Making Test for Screening Cognitive Impairment. J Am Geriatr Soc. 2018. 66(1): 92-99.

[24] Waheed W, Mirza N, Waheed MW, Malik A, Panagioti M. Developing and implementing guidelines on culturally adapting the Addenbrooke's cognitive examination version III (ACE-III): a qualitative illustration. BMC Psychiatry. 2020. 20(1): 492.

[25] Kokmen E, Naessens JM, Offord KP. A short test of mental status: description and preliminary results. Mayo Clin Proc. 1987. 62(4): 281-8.

[26] Tang-Wai DF, Knopman DS, Geda YE, et al. Comparison of the short test of mental status and the mini-mental state examination in mild cognitive impairment. Arch Neurol. 2003. 60(12): 1777-81.

[27] Kim JW, Byun MS, Sohn BK, et al. Clinical Dementia Rating Orientation Score as an Excellent Predictor of the Progression to Alzheimer's Disease in Mild Cognitive Impairment. Psychiatry Investig. 2017. 14(4): 420-426.

[28] Sousa A, Gomar JJ, Goldberg TE. Neural and behavioral substrates of disorientation in mild cognitive impairment and Alzheimer's disease. Alzheimers Dement (N Y). 2015. 1(1): 37-45.

[29] Guerrero-Berroa E, Luo X, Schmeidler J, et al. The MMSE orientation for time domain is a strong predictor of subsequent cognitive decline in the elderly. Int J Geriatr Psychiatry. 2009. 24(12): 1429-37.

[30] Choe YM, Lee BC, Choi IG, et al. MMSE Subscale Scores as Useful Predictors of AD Conversion in Mild Cognitive Impairment. Neuropsychiatr Dis Treat. 2020. 16: 1767-1775.

[31] Talboom JS, Håberg A, De Both MD, et al. Family history of Alzheimer's disease alters cognition and is modified by medical and genetic factors. Elife. 2019. 8.

[32] (ADI) ADI. World Alzheimer Report 2015-The Global Impact of Dementia. 2015. London. Alzheimer's Disease International (ADI).

[33] Dolgin E. How to defeat dementia. Nature. 2016. 539(7628): 156-158.

[34] James BD, Wilson RS, Boyle PA, Trojanowski JQ, Bennett DA, Schneider JA. TDP-43 stage, mixed pathologies, and clinical Alzheimer's-type dementia. Brain. 2016. 139(11): 2983.

[35] International AD. World Alzheimer Report 2016 (SUMMARY SHEET) .

[36] Anguera JA, Boccanfuso J, Rintoul JL, et al. Video game training enhances cognitive control in older adults. Nature. 2013. 501(7465): 97-101.

[37] Rebok GW, Ball K, Guey LT, et al. Ten-year effects of the advanced cognitive training for independent and vital elderly cognitive training trial on cognition and everyday functioning in older adults. J Am Geriatr Soc. 2014. 62(1): 16-24.

[38] Langa KM, Larson EB, Crimmins EM, et al. A Comparison of the Prevalence of Dementia in the United States in 2000 and 2012. JAMA Intern Med. 2017. 177(1): 51-58.

[39] Lourida I, Hannon E, Littlejohns TJ, et al. Association of Lifestyle and Genetic Risk With Incidence of Dementia. JAMA. 2019. 322(5): 430-437.

[40] Wolters FJ, Chibnik LB, Waziry R, et al. Twenty-seven-year time trends in dementia incidence in Europe and the United States: The

Alzheimer Cohorts Consortium. Neurology. 2020. 95(5): e519-e531.

[41] Heffernan M, Andrews G, Fiatarone Singh MA, et al. Maintain Your Brain: Protocol of a 3-Year Randomized Controlled Trial of a Personalized Multi-Modal Digital Health Intervention to Prevent Cognitive Decline Among Community Dwelling 55 to 77 Year Olds. J Alzheimers Dis. 2019. 70(s1): S221-S237.

[42] Sur S, Lin Z, Li Y, et al. Association of cerebrovascular reactivity and Alzheimer pathologic markers with cognitive performance. Neurology. 2020. 95(8): e962-e972.

[43] Wilcock D, Jicha G, Blacker D, et al. MarkVCID cerebral small vessel consortium: I. Enrollment, clinical, fluid protocols. Alzheimers Dement. 2021. 17(4): 704-715.

[44] Ashimatey BS, D'Orazio LM, Ma SJ, et al. Lower retinal capillary density in minimal cognitive impairment among older Latinx adults. Alzheimers Dement (Amst). 2020. 12(1): e12071.

[45] Eknoyan D, Hurley RA, Taber KH. The clock drawing task: common errors and functional neuroanatomy. J Neuropsychiatry Clin Neurosci. 2012. 24(3): 260-5.

[46] Cohen J, Penney DL, Davis R, et al. Digital Clock Drawing: differentiating "thinking" versus "doing" in younger and older adults with depression. J Int Neuropsychol Soc. 2014. 20(9): 920-8.

[47] Müller S, Preische O, Heymann P, Elbing U, Laske C. Increased Diagnostic Accuracy of Digital vs. Conventional Clock Drawing Test for Discrimination of Patients in the Early Course of Alzheimer's Disease from Cognitively Healthy Individuals. Front Aging Neurosci. 2017. 9: 101.

[48] Klaming L, Vlaskamp B. Non-dominant hand use increases completion time on part B of the Trail Making Test but not on part A. Behav Res Methods. 2018. 50(3): 1074-1087.

[49] Burns A, Gallagley A, Byrne J. Delirium. J Neurol Neurosurg Psychiatry. 2004. 75(3): 362-7.

SCREENING FALL RISKS IN COMMUNITY-DWELLING OLDER ADULTS WITH HIGH SENSITIVITY

Key points

- A battery (STABLE protocol) for fall prevention among community-dwelling older adults is introduced.
- The STABLE protocol consists of a modified version of STEADI, with high sensitivity and a more straightforward algorithm.
- Personality traits have an impact on the risk of falls, which may be partially reflected in the results of a clock-drawing test. A better effect of Tai Chi on fall prevention originates from the modulation of Tai Chi exercise to psychological, emotional, and personality traits.
- A modified single-leg stance is also proposed as an effective and efficient exercise for fall prevention.

Falls in elderly people cause unintentional injuries that may lead to serious consequences such as a hip fracture. The main causes of fall risks include biological, behavioral, environmental, and socioeconomic factors. Many tools have been developed to screen fall risks in hospitalized patients and community-dwelling older adults and provide interventions to prevent falls. However, several key issues still need to be addressed. First, it should be determined how sensitive a screening tool needs to be since low-sensitivity tools will leave out many elderly at risk of falls, and high-sensitivity methods should be adopted. In addition, a protocol should be able to target specific fall risk factors in biological, behavioral, environmental, and socioeconomic aspects in order to correct these factors. Moreover, approaches to effectively correct identified risk factors should be applied. Based on these considerations, we propose an evidence-based toolkit for screening elderly people at risk of falls in the community. Specific intervention methods are also provided.

No single recommended tool or brief approach can reliably identify older adults at increased risk for falls. It is not recommended to automatically perform an in-depth multifactorial risk assessment in conjunction with comprehensive management of identified risks to prevent falls in community-dwelling adults aged 65 years or older, because the likelihood of benefit is small [1].

Background

Falls are common causes of unintentional injuries in older adults and are a major or even the leading cause of injury-related morbidity and mortality among older people in many countries [2-4].

Falls are defined as inadvertently coming to rest on the ground, floor, or other lower level, excluding intentional changes in position to rest on furniture, wall, or other objects. The frequency of falls increases with age and frailty level, and falls may lead to serious conditions including hip fracture and traumatic brain injuries [5]. Thus, effective prevention of falls is urgent when population aging is becoming increasingly prominent in today's society in many countries.

Fall prevention needs to solve two problems: 1) to identify individuals with high fall risks, and 2) to effectively reduce the risks. The main factors of fall risks are classified into four categories: biological, behavioral, environmental, and socioeconomic factors [5]. Ideally, a predictive method is able to accurately assess the possibility of falls in older adults, and the results of the assessment can identify modifiable fall risk factors including balance deficits, gait abnormalities, environmental factors, and adverse effects of medication.

Various daily activities can lead to falls in the elderly [6] if the main risk factors are not identified and intervened. Note that restricting activity leads to more falls for older adults [7]. Therefore, an effective fall prevention protocol should identify factors leading to falls and then effectively correct these risk factors. The elderly needs to maintain safe, appropriate activities to slow down the decline of the musculoskeletal, cardiopulmonary, and other systems.

A solution to effectively assess individuals with a high risk of falls is needed for timely interventions. Currently, scales/questionnaires, behavioral tests, and instrumental tests are applied to measure fall risks.

Sensitivity is the percentage of persons with the disease/risk who are correctly identified by a test, and specificity is the percentage of persons without the disease/risk who are correctly excluded by the test. For fall prevention in the elderly, a higher or even overestimated sensitivity is preferred in that falls may lead to serious consequences such as hip fractures. A fall risk assessment tool should achieve a high enough sensitivity to identify as many elderly people with increased fall risks as possible. Fall prevention measures can then be timely applied. The sensitivityies of different tools are reviewed in the following sections.

Scales/questionnaires for hospitalized patients

Scales/questionnaires used to measure fall risks can be classified into two types, one for hospitalized patients and the other for community-dwelling older adults.

The Morse Fall Scale, the St. Thomas's Risk Assessment Tool in Falling Elderly Inpatients (STRATIFY) assessment tool, the Fall Risk Assessment Scale for the Elderly (FRASE), and the Johns Hopkins Fall Risk Assessment Tool are widely used scales to assess fall risks in hospitalized patients.

The Morse Fall Scale can be used to assess the likelihood of falling in hospital settings. It is a widely used scale whereas the developing process was seldom introduced in the literature. The scale was developed based on the data containing100 fallers and 100 randomly-selected non-fallers in a hospital. Fall risk factors of these hospitalized patients were examined and six items with a significance level of < 0.001 were chosen to form the scale: fall history within 3 months, secondary diagnosis, ambulatory levels, use of an intravenous apparatus/heparin lock, gait/transferring, and mental status. These six items can correctly classify 78% of the fall group [8].

The St. Thomas's Risk Assessment Tool in Falling Elderly Inpatients (STRATIFY) assessment tool is also a widely-used scale to briefly screen fall risks in hospitalized elderly patients. After comparing 116 cases and 116 controls, the scale was developed by using five items found to be independently associated with the risk of falling: fall history, impaired ability to transfer and walk, agitation, frequent toileting, and visual impairment. The scale was found to present a high sensitivity (92-93%) [9]. However, in a larger sample it only showed moderate (69%) to low (52%) sensitivity for patients admitted to geriatric wards and for patients ≥ 75 years old [10].

The Johns Hopkins Fall Risk Assessment Tool consists of seven risk factors: age, fall history, mobility, elimination, mental status changes, medication, and patient care equipment. These factors were selected from 8 previous scales [11]. The scale was revised after two years of practice; the content of each item and its weight were modified based on opinions from experts [12].

Similar to the Morse Fall Scale and STRATIFY, the Fall Risk Assessment Scale for the Elderly (FRASE) was designed to predict patients' risk of falling. It contains eight items: sex, sensory deficit, medical history, age, fall history, mobility, gait, and medication [13].

The Falls Risk Assessment Tool (FRAT) has three sections: Part 1, fall risk status; Part 2, risk factor checklist; and Part 3, action plan. Part 1 can be used as a falls risk screening test, which consists of four items, i.e., recent falls, medications, psychological status, and cognitive status. The item recent falls have a higher weight. The 4-item scale was found to have a sensitivity of 70.2% for predicting falls in hospitalized patients in the subacute and aged care populations[14]. A modified version for assessing fall risk for older people in the community was also developed, called the Falls Risk for Older People in the Community assessment (FROP-Com) tool. FROP-Com has a brief 3-item version for screening and a full version with 28 items (https://www.nari.net.au/frop-com). The FROP-Com has a sensitivity of 71.3% and specificity of 56.1% for fall prediction during 12 months, slightly better than the Timed Up and Go test and the functional reach test. The sensitivity/specificity of the 3-item version was not reported [15].

None of these widely-used scales demonstrates a high sensitivity (true positive rate). Note that even when a patient is randomly classified either in the fall group or in the control group, there will be a 50% probability of a correct classification [8]. Both FRASE and STRATIFY demonstrated poor sensitivity (50% or lower) in hip fracture patients [13]. The Morse scale presented a sensitivity of 83% in an acute care hospital [16]. Similar to the value of 78% reported in the original study [8]. Nevertheless, such a sensitivity (at the level of 80%) means about 20% of patients with fall risks failed to be recognized, and more patients with fall risks will be omitted if using tools with a lower sensitivity.

Why these meticulously designed scales cannot present high sensitivity? One possible reason is the heterogeneity of patients and internal/external fall risk factors in different hospitals and different areas/countries. For instance, studies using the same tool (the Johns Hopkins Fall Risk Assessment Tool) in different hospitals/areas presented various levels of sensitivity (26.5%, 62%, and 87.4%) [17-19]. The second possible reason is that some screening tools failed to include all the most important fall risk factors. To become a brief screening instrument, a scale cannot take in many items. However, whether or not a risk factor is included in a scale is contradictory in different tools, not to mention the weights of items in these scales. For example, the Morse Fall Scale does not assess visual impairments since this factor did not present a statistical difference between two groups during the development process of the scale [8], whereas STRATIFY contains this factor since visual impairment was found to be independently associated with a higher risk of falls in the studied sample [9]. The third reason may be the inappropriate application of the scales, especially for those having a relatively complex structure. In our experience in screening fall risks, when using a questionnaire for fall risk self-assessment by older adults [20], some subjects may not exactly understand the meaning of items in the questionnaire. Additionally, some medical staff may not accurately express the content of the items.

Then, what is the solution? To achieve higher sensitivity, one possible approach is to combine items from existing scales and allocate appropriate weights for each item. Another solution is to supplement external factors since these risk factors may account for 44-45% of contributory factors to falls [13, 21]. Adjusting the cut-off point is also a choice. For example, the Hendrich II Fall Risk Model presented a sensitivity of 78.72% when using a threshold score ≥ 5 but showed improvement in sensitivity (90.56%) at a lower cut-off score of ≥ 4 [7].

Scales/questionnaires for community-dwelling older adults

To assess fall risks in community-dwelling older adults, US Centers for Disease Control and Prevention adopts a short scale for fall risk assessment in its Stopping Elderly Accidents, Death & Injuries (STEADI) program [22]. The scale originates from a questionnaire for fall risk self-assessment in older adults that consists of 12 items [20]. During the development phase of the questionnaire, a comprehensive clinical evaluation of risks using the American/British Geriatrics Society guidelines was considered as the gold standard, including fall history, fear of falling, gait/balance, muscle weakness, incontinence, sensation and proprioception, depression, vision, and medications. Thirteen items were chosen first and the final 12 items and their weights were determined by using an iterative statistical approach.

The 12-item fall risk questionnaire covers major fall risk factors including:

- history of recent falls (item 1 "I have fallen in the last 6 months", or 12 months in the STEADI program),
- Afraid of falling (item 2 "I am worried about falling."),
- Balance deficiency (item 3 "Sometimes, I feel unsteady when I am walking" and item 4 "I steady myself by holding onto the furniture when walking at home."),
- Gait deficiency (item 5 "I use or have been advised to use a cane or walker to get around safely."),
- Muscle weakness (item 6 "I need to push with my hands to stand up from a chair." and item 7 "I have some trouble stepping up onto a curb."),
- Urinary incontinence (item 8 "I often have to rush to the toilet."),
- Abnormal peripheral sensation (item 9 "I have lost some feeling in my feet."), medications (item 10 "I take medicine that sometimes makes me feel light-headed or more tired than usual." and item 11 "I take medicine to help me sleep or improve my mood."),
- Depression (item 12 "I often feel sad or depressed.").

Item 1 (history of recent falls) and item 5 (gait deficiency) are weighted two points whereas each of the other items is given one point.

The final 12-item version was reported to present very high sensitivity (100%) and specificity (83.3%) [20]. But such sensitivity (100%) and specificity (83.3%) were acquired by comparing the scale and the abovementioned “gold standard” instead of verified in a longitudinal follow-up study.

A short version, i.e., the clinician’s 3 key questions, is also designed and used in the STEADI protocol, that is, asked by clinicians, “have you fallen in the last year, do you feel unsteady when standing or walking, and do you worry about falling?”. Compared to the 12-item questionnaire, using the three key questions can decrease the screening burden, but remarkably increased the number of detected high-risk subjects (281 vs. 170, from 773 outpatients) [23].

In a study with one-year follow-up, the clinician’s 3 key questions in the STEADI protocol demonstrated much better sensitivity than the 12-item fall risk questionnaire (93.8% vs. 77.7%) in community-dwelling older adults (Table 2 in [24]). Surprisingly, the clinician’s 3 key questions alone exhibited the highest sensitivity among all studied methods (the 12-item fall risk questionnaire, Timed Up and Go, 30-s-Chair Stand, and 4-Stage balance test) and their combinations in the STEADI protocol. Such a high sensitivity detected in a prospective study indicates that a short, easy-to-use scale can screen out the majority of community-dwelling elderly people at risk of falling.

The items of the clinician's 3 key questions are drawn from the 12-item questionnaire, whereas several differences exist. Firstly, the 3 key questions are asked by clinicians whereas the 12-item questionnaire is self-assessed by the older people. An experienced clinician understands the exact meaning of each item but the elderly may not. Thus, incorrect answers may be collected when using the 12-item questionnaire self-assessed by the elderly. Secondly, the items in the two methods have different weights. A "yes" to each item of the clinician's 3 key questions indicates at risk of falls; therefore, this tool is actually a combination of three one-question scales. Thirdly, the clinician's 3 key questions are very brief and straightforward, whereas the 12-item questionnaire has a longer content and more complex structure (the weight of two items is two points and the weight of other items is one point; a total score > 4 indicates the risk of falls). These differences can explain the high sensitivity of the 3 key questions.

Screening high-risk elderly and identifying fall risk factors with the STABLE protocol

When performing a study on fall prevention in the elderly (the STrategies and mechAnisms of community-Based falL prevention in the Elderly, STABLE; funded by the National Key R&D Program of China with Grant No. 2018YFC2001400), a protocol is applied based on the abovementioned evidence. It consists of several parts. First, the clinician's 3 key questions are used for screening. Afterwards, the 12-item questionnaire, the 3-level assessment of eyesight, and cognitive function measures are applied to identify fall risk factors in community-dwelling older adults.

The 12-item questionnaire can be adopted as a tool to identify fall risk factors performed by clinicians because the items in this tool reflect a broader scope of fall risks in comparison with the clinician's 3 key questions. Many common risk factors are shared by the 12-item questionnaire and other fall-screening scales. After screening fall risks by using the clinician's 3 key questions, a more extensive questionnaire can target specific problems which may lead to falls in older adults.

An item on visual acuity needs to be supplemented with the 12-item questionnaire. The original version of the 12-item self-assessment questionnaire included an item on visual acuity ("Because I don't see well, I have difficulty avoiding hazards in my path, such as tree roots or electrical cords."). However, only 15% of participants selected this item (i.e., stating the existence of poor vision), which is the smallest percentage among all 13 items. The self-reported poor vision did not agree well with results of visual acuity detected by the clinical examination, mainly due to false negatives: self-reported nonexistence of visual problem but clinically-identified positive vision impairment. As a result, the item on vision was excluded from the scale [20]. Nevertheless, 21 subjects (right eye 12 + left eye 9) among 40 participants were found to have poor visual acuity in the clinical assessment, presenting a higher ratio than many other factors (Table 1 in [20]). In fact, this finding supports the association between vision impairment and fall risks. The disagreement between a self-report and a clinical assessment may originate from the expression. "Avoiding hazards in my path such as tree roots or electrical cords" is a specific condition of vision impairment. Many subjects with vision problems chose to mark "no" possibly because they did not meet the specific difficulty in the item ("avoiding hazards in my path") although they did have vision problems. For example, the stairs may not be seen clearly in a dim environment by older people with weakened visual acuity, which results in falls. But this is not a condition of "hazards in my path such as tree roots or electrical cords". Additionally, the elderly may consider their visual problems as a natural aging process, and thus "I don't see well" is not a problem.

Here, a 3-level self-assessment of eyesight is recommended, i.e., Excellent and Good/Regular/Bad and Very Poor. This assessment is found to be associated with the occurrence of falls in a study involving 1593 elderly people [25]. The 3-level self-assessment is clear, simple, and easily understandable. When compared to those with excellent/good self-assessment, subjects reporting "Regular" and "Bad/Very Poor" eyesight had 52.0% and 96.0% more falls respectively. Thus, selecting "Excellent and Good" indicates a low risk of falls whereas selecting "Regular" or "Bad and Very Poor" is corresponding to increased fall risks; this dichotomic classification is consistent with the 12-item self-assessment questionnaire (i.e., "yes" or "no" to a given item). Note that many older adults consider functional degradation as a natural change caused by aging. Thus, a self-assessed "Regular" vision by the elderly often indicates varying degrees of vision loss and thus needs to be further investigated.

There is no item on cognitive function in the 12-item self-assessment questionnaire, because cognitive impairment cannot be reliably self-reported [20]. However, elderly people with cognitive impairment are at increased risk of falls, and therefore cognitive assessment, particularly executive function, should be integrated into fall risk screening [26].

Cognitive impairment together with physical frailty results in a greater risk for fall-related fractures than cognitive impairment or physical frailty alone [27]. Note that different cognitive domains may have various impacts on fall risks. In elderly people, worse executive function is found to be associated with increased single and recurrent falls [28]. The cognitive function modifies the effect of physiological function on the risk of multiple falls [29] and can predict falls [30], whereas memory was not related to either single or recurrent falls [28] but associated with less mobility decline among non-fallers [31].

Motor function tests

There are several widely-used motor function tests to screen fall risks. Additionally, some tools such as the Hendrich II Fall Risk Model and the STEADI Tool Kit consist of both scale/questionnaire and motor function tests.

The Berg Balance Scale (BBS) is often used in clinical practice to predict falls in older adults. It measures steady-state and dynamic postural control, including unsupported sitting, sitting to standing, standing to sitting, transfers, unsupported standing, standing with eyes closed, standing with feet together, Tandem standing, standing on one leg, turning trunk (feet fixed), retrieving objects from the floor, turning 360 degrees, stool stepping, reaching forward while standing [32, 33]. Some of these items are used in other tests. The evidence of using the Berg Balance Scale alone to predict falls is lacking [34]. For example, when using the Berg Balance Scale as a dichotomous scale with a threshold of < or =45, it was insufficient to identify the majority of people at risk of falls (sensitivities of 25% and 45% for any fall and multiple falls) [35].

The STEADI protocol and the Short Physical Performance Battery (SPPB)[36] assess lower limb strength, balance, and walking ability with several motion paradigms: the feet together in the side-by-side, semi-tandem, and tandem positions, chair standing and walking speed (Timed 8-Foot Walk or Timed Up and Go). The walking speed is not tested in the Berg Balance Scale.

The Tinetti gait and balance assessment is a more comprehensive examination than the STEADI and SPPB. It can differentiate recurrent fallers and those who fell once or not at all [37]. Compared to a single fall, multiple falls put patients at a higher risk of injury. There are a few unique paradigms adopted in the Tinetti assessment in comparison with the STEADI/SPPB, including walking at rapid speed, immediate standing balance (first 5 sec), a Romberg test with nudge and/or eyes closed, and turning 360 degrees (a complete circle). These motor tasks are challengeable (rapid walking, immediate standing balance, and Romberg test with eyes closed) or targeted (turning a complete circle) and thus more likely to detect functional deficits.

When screening older adults at risk of falls in the community, some seniors were found to present immediate standing balance deficits during testing such as a semi-tandem, tandem position, or a one-legged stance. These individuals may exhibit a more stable balance control when they perform the task again, thereby presenting a learning effect. Falls are biomechanical events during which various factors destabilize the body's alignment to cause inadvertently falling down to the ground, floor, or other lower levels. When facing such an event, an instant response is crucial to maintain/restore balance. Thus, an immediate response to a standing test is sensitive to revealing functional deficits. For example, during the first trial (the immediate response) of the Tandem (Heel-Toe) stance, non-fallers and fallers exhibit a difference of around 20 s (median value), whereas the difference during the best trial (practice effect) is less than 4 s [38]. For a single-leg stance test, during the first 5 s the force variability decreased significantly more in the young group than in the elderly, resulting in a lower force variability level in this period in the young group [39].

If a screening protocol does not clearly show whether an immediate response or a more stable response after practice during a balance test should be assessed, the results of the test may record either condition and will not be consistent.

A Romberg test with eyes closed is more likely to detect impaired balance control than the test in an eyes open condition. Moreover, a positive Romberg test with eyes closed can indicate proprioception disorders if no somatosensory test is applied. Note that proprioceptive senses, particularly limb position and movement, deteriorate with aging and are associated with an increased risk of falls in the elderly [40].

Turning 360 degrees is a test that can differentiate recurrent fallers and single- or non-fallers [37]. Both walking-and-turning and standing-and-turning have been proven to lead to falls in the elderly [6, 41, 42]. A Timed Up and Go test includes a rotation of the body, but turning a complete circle is more specific for identifying instability when the body rotates. Compared to gait speed, the duration alone of the Timed Up and Go test did not present a better predictive ability for falls [43], possibly due to either the "dilution" effect of gait speed on the entire test or lacking a sensitive assessment for turning components in the Timed Up and Go test. Therefore, a test specific to turning is needed.

The Tinetti assessment has better test-retest, discriminative and predictive validities for assessing fall risks than the Timed Up and Go test (TUG), One-leg stand test, and functional reach test [37]. However, its pooled sensitivity from two studies was found to be 0.68, which is not a high value [44]. Note that only several items of the Tinetti assessment were associated with falling [37]. Therefore, although the Tinetti assessment adopts several motor paradigms which recreate fall situations [37] and examines specific balance functional defects, other items in this tool impair its sensitivity for predicting falls.

None of the commonly-used motor function tests present sensitivity higher than 90% [44]. Two possible reasons exist. On the one hand, falls are caused by multiple factors, which cannot be reflected by assessing motor function alone. On the other hand, many behavioral tests consist of items sensitive to fall risks and those insensitive for predicting falls in the elderly.

Thus, it may be better to use sensitive items to target specific balance function deficits in comparison with using a motor function test to screen fall risks. A video-recorded study on the circumstances of falls emphasized two factors, the causes of falls and activities leading to falls. Causes of falls were classified into seven types, 1) incorrect transfer or shift of body weight, 2) trip or stumble, 3) hit or bump, 4) loss of support with external objects, 5) collapse or loss of consciousness, 6) slip, and 7) could not tell. Activities leading to falls were classified into 11 types, 1) walking forward, 2) standing quietly, 3) sitting down or lowering, 4) initiation of walking, 5) getting up or rising, 6) walking backward/sideways, 7) walking and turning, 8) standing and turning, 9) seated or wheeling in wheelchairs, 10) standing and reaching, and 11) could not tell [6]. These scenarios where a fall happens need to be considered as items.

The adopted items should be challenging enough because a balance function assessment measures anticipatory postural adjustments whereas a fall in the elderly is often caused by unexpected events. Under such conditions, preventing a fall needs a better balance function, which cannot be detected by a balance test without sufficient difficulty/challeng.

The STABLE protocol for screening fall risks in community-dwelling older adults

The STABLE protocol aims to provide a short, easy-to-use tool with high sensitivity (> 90%) to screen out community-dwelling older people at risk of falls. It is a toolkit consisting of three parts/levels.

The first level aims to screen out the elderly at risk of falls by using the 3 key questions asked by clinicians:

- Have you fallen in the last year;
- Do you feel unsteady when standing or walking;
- Do you worry about falling?

A "yes" to any of the three items indicates at risk of falls.

For older people identified to have an increased risk of falls by the first level screening, the second and third parts should be performed to identify specific risk factors.

The second level contains a series of items to identify fall risk factors:

① The 12-item questionnaire, to examine the history of recent falls, afraid of falling, balance deficiency, gait deficiency, muscle weakness, urinary incontinence, abnormal peripheral sensation, medications, and depression:

- Have you fallen in the past 12 months?
- Recently, do you use or have been advised by medical professionals to use walking aids (such as a cane, crutch, or walker) for walking safely?
- Do you feel unsteady during walking?
- Do you steady yourself by holding onto furniture or wall when walking at home?
- Are you worried about falling?
- Do you need to push with your hands to stand up from a chair?
- Do you have any trouble stepping up onto a curb?
- Do you often have to rush to the toilet due to incontinence?
- Do you have lost some feeling in your feet?
- Do you take medicine that sometimes makes you feel light-headed or more tired than usual?
- Do you take medicine to help you sleep or improve your mood?
- Do you often feel sad or depressed?

Each positive answer indicates corresponding clinical disorders.

② The 3-level assessment of eyesight: Excellent and Good/Regular/Bad and Very Poor. Choosing "Regular" or "Bad/Very Poor" indicates fall risks due to impaired visual acuity.

- How do you feel about your vision, Excellent and Good, Regular, or Bad and Very Poor?

Choosing "Regular", or "Bad and Very Poor" indicates impaired visual acuity that may need intervention.

③ The Quick-Cog scale, to evaluate cognitive function. A basic version assesses executive function and memory, which can be completed within 3 min (a full version examines more cognitive domains and can be completed within 15 min). The basic version consists of three parts:

- Immediate recall (assessing memory)
- Clock drawing (assessing executive function)
- Delayed recall (assessing memory)

Better executive function, but not attention, memory, or visuospatial function, was associated with less decline in mobility among fallers. Better memory function, but not other cognitive domains, was associated with less mobility decline among non-fallers [31].

Personality traits can be observed when testing clock drawing. Two manifestations are inconsistent with the conscientiousness trait: the elderly begin to draw a circle before the instruction is completed, or the drawn circle is not very round though the upper limb motor function is fine.

The third level evaluates balance, gait, strength, endurance, and proprioception. It consists of the following items:

- Timed Up and Go test at the usual speed
- Timed Up and Go test at the fastest (but safe) speed
- 30-Second Chair Stand Test
- Parallel stance (side-by-side stand) with eyes open
- Parallel stance (side-by-side stand) with eyes closed
- Semi-tandem stance (instep of one foot touching the big toe of the other foot)
- Tandem (Heel-Toe) stance (each foot in front once)
- Single leg stance (each foot once)
- Turning 360 degrees (a complete circle; clockwise, counterclockwise)

*The duration of the single leg stance is similar for fallers and non-fallers (around 10 s) [38].

* The elderly (aged 60 to 89 years) may maintain the Tandem (Heel-Toe) stance longer than 60 s (50% of the fallers and 67% of the non-fallers were able to reach 60 s and a longer duration was not tested) [38].

The aim of this level is not to estimate the risk of falls but examine which function of the body is impaired. The items are selected mainly from two brief methods, the SPPB and STEADI protocol. Referring to the Tinetti assessment, several additional items are supplemented: 1) the proprioception is examined by using Romberg's test, i.e., the feet together in the side-by-side position, the eyes open and then closed for 10 s. The eyes-closed condition is not examined by the SPPB and STEADI protocol but it directly corresponds to proprioceptive deficits of the feet. 2) A fast Timed Up and Go test is adopted. That is, after performing a Timed Up and Go test with a usual speed, a subject is required to complete the test as fast as possible. The fast test is more challenging in order to magnify functional deficits. 3) Due to the unexpectedness of the occurrence of falls, the tandem (Heel-Toe) stance is examined with each foot in front separately, and turning 360 degrees clockwise and counterclockwise should be assessed separately.

The immediate response should be used to assess the performance because a fall often occurs unexpectedly and instant response is critical to maintaining balance in this condition. For each item, the elderly are considered to have functional deficits if a good performance can be achieved after practice but the immediate response is unsteady. Such a learning effect indicates a potential to improve balance function after training. More or longer practice/attempts to achieve a good performance imply a weaker potential.

All contents of the STABLE protocol need to be administrated by a clinician via a one-to-one test or a group test. A self-assessment may lead to inaccurate results.

Fall prevention

Based on risk factors identified by using the STABLE protocol, targeted interventions should be used.

Additionally, reducing environmental risk factors should be emphasized, e.g., increasing the amount of light (especially at night), avoiding walking on slippery surfaces, keeping the floor clear, and changing structural hazards such as a broken step reduces fall risks [45].

During community screening, we notice that some active, incautious older adults suffer falls. A careless person may often overlook risks in the surrounding environment and thus is more likely to fall. The Australia guide to preventing falls also emphasizes "Don't rush, take your time" for the elderly in public places [45]. Lower conscientiousness (organized, responsible, hardworking, and not careless) and higher neuroticism (moody, worrying, nervous, and not calm) are found to increase the risk of falls [46]. Taken together, personality traits, i.e., an individual's characteristic ways of thinking, feeling, and behaving have an impact on the risk of falls.

Personality traits of an individual can be observed when tested with the STABLE protocol, e.g., whether the subject follows the instructions well, or the performance of the clock drawing test.

Compared to stretching, multimodal exercise (including aerobic conditioning, strength, balance, and flexibility activities) and Tai Chi (i.e., Tai Ji Quan) can reduce the incidence of falls among community-dwelling older adults at high risk of falling. Additionally, Tai Chi is more effective than multimodal exercise [47]. The adopted Tai Chi is a practice focused on controlled exercises with synchronized breathing, including the center of gravity displacement using a dynamic interplay of stabilizing and self-induced destabilizing postural actions. The postural actions involve unilateral weight-bearing and weight-shifting movements, trunk and pelvic rotation, ankle sway, and eye-head-hand movements [48].

The benefit of Tai Chi on fall prevention is attributed to several reasons, including enhanced balance control of the elderly by practicing self-induced destabilizing postural actions, increased muscle strength and endurance via weight bearing [49], improved flexibility acquired during the slow, continuous movement similar to dynamic stretching [50]. Tai Chi can improve cognitive performance (executive function, measured by the Trail Making Test) [51, 52]. Notably, worse executive function is associated with increased single and recurrent falls in the elderly [28] and better executive function is associated with a less decline in mobility among fallers [31]. Tai Chi intervention also improves the proprioception of the knee and ankle [53] and sleep quality [54], which benefit fall prevention. Additionally, Tai Chi exercise increases parasympathetic activity, decreases sympathetic activity [50], improves mood, and decreases stress, anxiety, and depression [55, 56]. The slow, precise, controlled movement during Tai Chi exercise tends to build an enduring, calm, cautious behavior consistent with a conscientiousness personality trait, thereby reducing fall risks.

The improved balance, strength, and flexibility are common training effects of Tai Chi and the multimodal exercise. A better effect of Tai Chi on fall prevention originates from the modulation of Tai Chi exercise to psychological, emotional, and personality traits.

The single-leg stance is a simple postural exercise. A short period of single-leg stance exercise (eyes closed, 10 x 64-second, alternately standing on the left or right foot) can improve two-leg postural control [57]. Actually, only one or two trials can prolong the duration of a single-leg stance, whether with eyes open or closed [38]. A 6-month single leg stance exercise with open eyes for 1 min three times per day can reduce the incidence of falls in young and older adults (37 to 102 years, patients or community-dwelling people) [58]. In elderly people ≥75 years of age, this intervention can improve independence in daily living in addition to reducing fall risks [59]. In women aged ≥ 70 years, such exercise can increase hip total bone mineral density [60]. Theoretically, performing the single-leg stance for 1 minute provides a load equivalent to that from about 1 hour of walking [61]. Note that bone mass can be increased by a strength exercise using high-load low repetitions but not by an endurance exercise using low-load high repetitions [62]. Thus, it is also an efficient weight-bearing exercise to delay the decrease in bone density. Higher-impact physical activity is associated with the maintenance of bone mineral density in the elderly, but cannot reduce incident falls [63]. These findings indicate that the single-leg stance is unique for the effects on maintaining bone density and reducing fall incidence.

Here, we introduce a modified single-leg stance following the principle of Tai Chi. During the single-leg stance exercise, the lifting leg moves in different directions, i.e., raising-lowering, front-back, abduction-adduction, and rotating clockwise/ counterclockwise centered at the hip joint. The individual performs movements in a slow, precise, controlled, continuous manner, and perceives changes in the center of gravity. The arms are also raised and lowered (shoulder abduction-adduction) when the legs are not moving during a one-leg stance. Every movement can be performed for 1 min, three times per day. Eyes-closed practice can enhance challenges.

The proposed single-leg stance exercise preserves the features of the conventional one-leg stance (i.e., high intensity within a short period) but has a higher difficulty. In addition, it has the advantage of Tai Chi: moving the body in a gentle, flowing manner and carefully maintaining/feeling changes in the center of gravity may help to shape a calm and cautious behavior in consistent with a conscientiousness personality trait.

The single-leg stance is also a very efficient body-weight bearing exercise. For elderly people, standing on one leg for one minute leads to a load on the femoral head equaling to walking for one hour (exactly speaking, 53.3 minutes) [64].

Conclusion

This chapter introduces the STABLE protocol for fall prevention among community-dwelling older adults. The STABLE protocol consists of a very brief screening method with high sensitivity, and a group of questions and cognitive and motor tests to identify specific risk factors. In addition to intervening detected risk factors of falls, reducing environmental risk factors should not be omitted.

Tai Chi is more effective than multimodal exercise (including aerobic conditioning, strength, balance, and flexibility activities) to reduce fall incidence in the elderly. The core elements of Tai Chi are introduced. Besides enhancing balance, strength, and flexibility, the mode of performing movement during Tai Chi may shape a conscientiousness personality trait, thereby resulting in a special benefit. A modified single-leg stance is also proposed to provide a convenient but high-efficient exercise, which can be used everywhere, every time in every day.

References

[1] Moyer VA, U.S. Preventive Services Task Force. Prevention of falls in community-dwelling older adults: U.S. Preventive Services Task Force recommendation statement. Ann Intern Med. 2012; 157: 197-204.

[2] Hagiya H, Koyama T, Zamami Y, et al. Fall-related mortality trends in older Japanese adults aged ≥65 years: a nationwide observational study. BMJ Open. 2019; 9: e033462.

[3] Zhang L, Ding Z, Qiu L, Li A. Falls and risk factors of falls for urban and rural community-dwelling older adults in China. BMC Geriatr. 2019; 19: 379.

[4] Web-based Injury Statistics Query and Reporting System (WISQARS) website ,2019.

[5] Organization WH. WHO Global Report on Falls Prevention in Older Age. 2007. 1st. France. World Health Organization.

[6] Robinovitch SN, Feldman F, Yang Y, et al. Video capture of the circumstances of falls in elderly people residing in long-term care: an observational study. Lancet. 2013; 381: 47-54.

[7] Hendrich AL, Bufalino A, Groves C. Validation of the Hendrich II Fall Risk Model: The imperative to reduce modifiable risk factors. Appl Nurs Res. 2020; 53: 151243.

[8] Morse JM, Morse RM, Tylko SJ. Development of a Scale to Identify the Fall-Prone Patient. Canadian Journal on Aging / La Revue canadienne du vieillissement. 1989; 8: 366-377.

[9] Oliver D, Britton M, Seed P, Martin FC, Hopper AH. Development and evaluation of evidence based risk assessment tool (STRATIFY)

to predict which elderly inpatients will fall: case-control and cohort studies. BMJ. 1997; 315: 1049-53.

[10] Milisen K, Staelens N, Schwendimann R, et al. Fall prediction in inpatients by bedside nurses using the St. Thomas's Risk Assessment Tool in Falling Elderly Inpatients (STRATIFY) instrument: a multicenter study. J Am Geriatr Soc. 2007; 55: 725-33.

[11] Poe SS, Cvach MM, Gartrelu DG, Radzik BR, Joy TL. An evidence-based approach to fall risk assessment, prevention, and management: lessons learned. J Nurs Care Qual. 2005; 20: 107-16; quiz 117-8.

[12] Poe SS, Cvach M, Dawson PB, Straus H, Hill EE. The Johns Hopkins Fall Risk Assessment Tool: postimplementation evaluation. J Nurs Care Qual. 2007; 22: 293-8.

[13] Jester R, Wade S, Henderson K. A pilot investigation of the efficacy of falls risk assessment tools and prevention strategies in an elderly hip fracture population. Journal of Orthopaedic Nursing. 2005; 9: 27.

[14] Stapleton C, Hough P, Oldmeadow L, Bull K, Hill K, Greenwood K. Four-item fall risk screening tool for subacute and residential aged care: The first step in fall prevention. Australas J Ageing. 2009; 28: 139-43.

[15] Russell MA, Hill KD, Blackberry I, Day LM, Dharmage SC. The reliability and predictive accuracy of the falls risk for older people in the community assessment (FROP-Com) tool. Age Ageing. 2008; 37: 634-9.

[16] O'Connell B, Myers H. The sensitivity and specificity of the Morse Fall Scale in an acute care setting. J Clin Nurs. 2002; 11: 134-6.

[17] Klinkenberg WD, Potter P. Validity of the Johns Hopkins Fall Risk Assessment Tool for Predicting Falls on Inpatient Medicine Services. J Nurs Care Qual. 2017; 32: 108-113.

[18] Kim KS, Kim JA, Choi YK, et al. A comparative study on the validity of fall risk assessment scales in korean hospitals. Asian Nurs Res (Korean Soc Nurs Sci). 2011; 5: 28-37.

[19] Poe SS, Dawson PB, Cvach M, et al. The Johns Hopkins Fall Risk Assessment Tool: A Study of Reliability and Validity. J Nurs Care Qual. 2018; 33: 10-19.

[20] Rubenstein LZ, Vivrette R, Harker JO, Stevens JA, Kramer BJ. Validating an evidence-based, self-rated fall risk questionnaire (FRQ) for older adults. J Safety Res. 2011; 42: 493-9.

[21] Tinetti ME, Speechley M, Ginter SF. Risk factors for falls among elderly persons living in the community. N Engl J Med. 1988; 319: 1701-7.

[22] Bergen G, Shakya I. CDC STEADI: Evaluation Guide for Older Adult Clinical Fall Prevention Programs. 2019ed. USA:US Centers for Disease Control and Prevention,2019.

[23] Eckstrom E, Parker EM, Lambert GH, Winkler G, Dowler D, Casey CM. Implementing STEADI in Academic Primary Care to Address Older Adult Fall Risk. Innov Aging. 2017; 1: igx028.

[24] Loonlawong S, Limroongreungrat W, Rattananupong T, Kittipimpanon K, Saisanan Na Ayudhaya W, Jiamjarasrangsi W. Predictive validity of the Stopping Elderly Accidents, Deaths & Injuries (STEADI) program fall risk screening algorithms among

community-dwelling Thai elderly. BMC Med. 2022； 20: 78.

[25] Nunes BP, de Oliveira Saes M, Siqueira FV, et al. Falls and self-assessment of eyesight among elderly people: a population-based study in a south Brazilian municipality. Arch Gerontol Geriatr. 2014； 59: 131-5.

[26] Zhang W, Low LF, Schwenk M, Mills N, Gwynn JD, Clemson L. Review of Gait, Cognition, and Fall Risks with Implications for Fall Prevention in Older Adults with Dementia. Dement Geriatr Cogn Disord. 2019； 48: 17-29.

[27] Tsutsumimoto K, Doi T, Makizako H, et al. Cognitive Frailty is Associated with Fall-Related Fracture among Older People. J Nutr Health Aging. 2018； 22: 1216-1220.

[28] Holtzer R, Friedman R, Lipton RB, Katz M, Xue X, Verghese J. The relationship between specific cognitive functions and falls in aging. Neuropsychology. 2007； 21: 540-8.

[29] Martin KL, Blizzard L, Srikanth VK, et al. Cognitive function modifies the effect of physiological function on the risk of multiple falls--a population-based study. J Gerontol A Biol Sci Med Sci. 2013； 68: 1091-7.

[30] Saverino A, Waller D, Rantell K, Parry R, Moriarty A, Playford ED. The Role of Cognitive Factors in Predicting Balance and Fall Risk in a Neuro-Rehabilitation Setting. PLoS One. 2016； 11: e0153469.

[31] Hughes TF, Beer JC, Jacobsen E, Ganguli M, Chang CH, Rosano C. Executive function predicts decline in mobility after a fall: The MYHAT study. Exp Gerontol. 2020； 137: 110948.

[32] Berg K, Wood-Dauphine S, Williams JI, Gayton D. Measuring

balance in the elderly: preliminary development of an instrument. Physiotherapy CanadaPhysiotherapy Canada. 1989；41: 304.

[33] Lajoie Y, Gallagher SP. Predicting falls within the elderly community: comparison of postural sway, reaction time, the Berg balance scale and the Activities-specific Balance Confidence (ABC) scale for comparing fallers and non-fallers. Arch Gerontol Geriatr. 2004；38: 11-26.

[34] Lima CA, Ricci NA, Nogueira EC, Perracini MR. The Berg Balance Scale as a clinical screening tool to predict fall risk in older adults: a systematic review. Physiotherapy. 2018；104: 383-394.

[35] Muir SW, Berg K, Chesworth B, Speechley M. Use of the Berg Balance Scale for predicting multiple falls in community-dwelling elderly people: a prospective study. Phys Ther. 2008；88: 449-59.

[36] Guralnik JM, Simonsick EM, Ferrucci L, et al. A short physical performance battery assessing lower extremity function: association with self-reported disability and prediction of mortality and nursing home admission. J Gerontol. 1994；49: M85-94.

[37] Tinetti ME, Williams TF, Mayewski R. Fall risk index for elderly patients based on number of chronic disabilities. Am J Med. 1986；80: 429-34.

[38] Heitmann DK, Gossman MR, Shaddeau SA, Jackson JR. Balance performance and step width in noninstitutionalized, elderly, female fallers and nonfallers. Phys Ther. 1989；69: 923-31.

[39] Jonsson E, Seiger A, Hirschfeld H. One-leg stance in healthy young and elderly adults: a measure of postural steadiness. Clin Biomech (Bristol, Avon). 2004；19: 688-94.

[40] Proske U, Gandevia SC. The proprioceptive senses: their roles in signaling body shape, body position and movement, and muscle force. Physiol Rev. 2012; 92: 1651-97.

[41] Hayes WC, Myers ER, Robinovitch SN, Van Den Kroonenberg A, Courtney AC, McMahon TA. Etiology and prevention of age-related hip fractures. Bone. 1996; 18: 77S-86S.

[42] Noury N, Fleury A, Rumeau P, et al. Fall detection--principles and methods. Annu Int Conf IEEE Eng Med Biol Soc. 2007; 2007: 1663-6.

[43] Viccaro LJ, Perera S, Studenski SA. Is timed up and go better than gait speed in predicting health, function, and falls in older adults. J Am Geriatr Soc. 2011; 59: 887-92.

[44] Park SH. Tools for assessing fall risk in the elderly: a systematic review and meta-analysis. Aging Clin Exp Res. 2018; 30: 1-16.

[45] Australia Co. Don't Fall For It- A guide to preventing falls for older people. 2011. 2011. Australia. Department of Health and Ageing. 1-35.

[46] Canada B, Stephan Y, Sutin AR, Terracciano A. Personality and Falls Among Older Adults: Evidence From a Longitudinal Cohort. J Gerontol B Psychol Sci Soc Sci. 2020; 75: 1905-1910.

[47] Li F, Harmer P, Fitzgerald K, et al. Effectiveness of a Therapeutic Tai Ji Quan Intervention vs a Multimodal Exercise Intervention to Prevent Falls Among Older Adults at High Risk of Falling: A Randomized Clinical Trial. JAMA Intern Med. 2018; 178: 1301-1310.

[48] Li F. Transforming traditional Tai Ji Quan techniques into integrative movement therapy-Tai Ji Quan: Moving for Better

Balance. J Sport Health Sci. 2014; 3: 9-15.

[49] Yang F, Liu W. Biomechanical mechanism of Tai-Chi gait for preventing falls: A pilot study. J Biomech. 2020; 105: 109769.

[50] Audette JF, Jin YS, Newcomer R, Stein L, Duncan G, Frontera WR. Tai Chi versus brisk walking in elderly women. Age Ageing. 2006; 35: 388-93.

[51] Nguyen MH, Kruse A. A randomized controlled trial of Tai chi for balance, sleep quality and cognitive performance in elderly Vietnamese. Clin Interv Aging. 2012; 7: 185-90.

[52] Sungkarat S, Boripuntakul S, Kumfu S, Lord SR, Chattipakorn N. Tai Chi Improves Cognition and Plasma BDNF in Older Adults With Mild Cognitive Impairment: A Randomized Controlled Trial. Neurorehabil Neural Repair. 2018; 32: 142-149.

[53] Hu X, Lai Z, Wang L. Effects of Taichi exercise on knee and ankle proprioception among individuals with knee osteoarthritis. Res Sports Med. 2020; 28: 268-278.

[54] Du S, Dong J, Zhang H, et al. Taichi exercise for self-rated sleep quality in older people: a systematic review and meta-analysis. Int J Nurs Stud. 2015; 52: 368-79.

[55] Zheng S, Kim C, Lal S, Meier P, Sibbritt D, Zaslawski C. The Effects of Twelve Weeks of Tai Chi Practice on Anxiety in Stressed But Healthy People Compared to Exercise and Wait-List Groups-A Randomized Controlled Trial. J Clin Psychol. 2018; 74: 83-92.

[56] Huston P, McFarlane B. Health benefits of tai chi: What is the evidence. Can Fam Physician. 2016; 62: 881-890.

[57] Burdet C, Vuillerme N, Rougier PR. How performing a repetitive

one-legged stance modifies two-legged postural control. J Strength Cond Res. 2011; 25: 2911-8.

[58] Sakamoto K, Nakamura T, Hagino H, et al. Effects of unipedal standing balance exercise on the prevention of falls and hip fracture among clinically defined high-risk elderly individuals: a randomized controlled trial. J Orthop Sci. 2006; 11: 467-72.

[59] Sakamoto K, Endo N, Harada A, et al. Why not use your own body weight to prevent falls? A randomized, controlled trial of balance therapy to prevent falls and fractures for elderly people who can stand on one leg for ≤15 s. J Orthop Sci. 2013; 18: 110-20.

[60] Sakai A, Oshige T, Zenke Y, Yamanaka Y, Nagaishi H, Nakamura T. Unipedal standing exercise and hip bone mineral density in postmenopausal women: a randomized controlled trial. J Bone Miner Metab. 2010; 28: 42-8.

[61] Sakamoto K, Sugimoto F, Sato Y, Fujimaki E, Tashiro Y. Dynamic Flamingo Therapy for Prevention of Femoral Neck Osteoporosis and Fractures. The Showa University Journal of Medical Sciences. 1999; 11: 247.

[62] Kerr D, Morton A, Dick I, Prince R. Exercise effects on bone mass in postmenopausal women are site-specific and load-dependent. J Bone Miner Res. 1996; 11: 218-25.

[63] Ng CA, Scott D, Seibel MJ, et al. Higher-Impact Physical Activity Is Associated With Maintenance of Bone Mineral Density But Not Reduced Incident Falls or Fractures in Older Men: The Concord Health and Aging in Men Project. J Bone Miner Res. 2021; 36: 662-672.

[64] Kelzo SAKAMOTO, Futoshl SUGIMOTO, Yoshisada SATO, Etsuo FUJIMAKI and Y Oshlhlsa TASHIRO. Dynamic Flamingo Therapy for Prevention of Femoral Neck Osteoporosis and Fractures.Part 1: Theoretical Background. Showa Univ J Med Sci. 1999; 11: 247-254.

SCREENING, EVALUATION, AND TREATMENT FOR DYSPHAGIA

Key points

- How should dysphagia screening be performed?
- Why is sequential water swallowing test needed?
- Besides a decrease, a post-swallowing increase in SpO2 may indicate abnormality.
- What is the 3-ortho principle for helping beginners to complete FEES insertion?
- What types of the dye should be used in FEES?
- Oropharyngeal electrical-vibration stimulation is better than electrical stimulation or vibration stimulation alone.
- How to perform a balloon-catheter dilation for treating UES dysfunction?

Dysphagia (also known as difficulty in swallowing) is a common and serious problem for many diseases including stroke, Parkinson's disease, traumatic brain injury, [1], Alzheimer's disease [2], and mental illness [3]. Dysphagia causes serious complications including malnutrition, weight loss, aspiration pneumonia, premature mortality, and asphyxia, and affects people of all ages [4] [5]. Notably, approximately of 9/10 community-acquired pneumonia patients suffer from dysphagia [6].

In this chapter, a feasible protocol for screening dysphagia in the community and hospitalized patients is proposed. Unique explanations for values of pulse oximetry and wet voice during dysphagia screening are provided.

Based on a 3D understanding of dysphagia that incorporates VFSS, FEES, and anatomy, NME-vibration stimulation is introduced as a very effective method to activate swallowing function.

Physiology and pathophysiology of swallow

Swallowing is the process to move materials from the oral cavity to the stomach. Healthy adults swallow approximately 600 times in 24 hours. 150 of these swallows are related to feeding and the remains are unconscious swallows primarily for the clearance of saliva. During sleep, healthy subjects swallow around 4 times per hour [7].

A swallow can be divided into three phases, i.e., the oral, pharyngeal, and esophageal phases base on the locations of the transported material. The swallowed liquid/solid material is called the "bolus". During the oral phase, a bolus is transported from the oral cavity to the pharyngeal aperture. During the pharyngeal phase, the bolus passes through the cricopharyngeal region, which is the junction between the pharyngeal phase and the esophageal phase. In the esophageal phase, the bolus enters the esophagus at the cricopharyngeal region and finally arrives at the stomach through the lower esophagus sphincter.

During the pharyngeal phase, the inlet of the airway is closed, which occurs along with the opening of the entrance of the esophagus, i.e., the upper esophageal sphincter. This mechanism is crucial for avoiding food from entering the airway. The key to a normal pharyngeal protection mechanism is the timely and adequate closure of the airway, which includes closure of the larynx and downward movement of the epiglottis (epiglottis retroflexion) to cover the larynx inlet. Note that an individual can be free of penetration/aspiration if the larynx is adequately and timely closed even when the epiglottis is absent, that is, the protective effect of the epiglottis is not essential for a safe swallow. During swallow, the upper part of the larynx is closed at two levels, i.e., the laryngeal inlet and the vocal cords. Swallow-induced vocal cord adduction occurs prior to the onset of tongue base movement, superior hyoid movement, submental myoelectrical activity, pharyngeal peristalsis, UES opening, and laryngeal inlet closure. Additionally, the vocal cord abduction is the last one among all these events during swallow [7]. These findings indicate that the larynx closure, especially the vocal cord abduction, is a key protective factor during swallow. FEES can visualize the sequential actions of vocal cord adduction and then the laryngeal inlet closure during swallow, which forms double barriers to prevent food/liquid/saliva from entering the lower respiratory tract. Breaking through the first barrier (the laryngeal inlet) is called penetration, and breaking through the second barrier (the vocal cords) is called aspiration. Aryepiglotticus, oblique arytenoid, and transverse arytenoid form the sphincter to close the laryngeal inlet [8, 9].

Airway invasion of swallowed materials may cause serious consequences, including penetration, aspiration, and asphyxia. Penetration is the entrance of swallowed material into the larynx that does not pass below the vocal cords. Aspiration is defined as the passage of material below the level of the vocal cords. An 8-point scale can be used to quantify the depth of airway invasion and whether or not material entering the airway is expelled [10].

Patients and healthy subjects may or may not cough in response to food/liquid entering the laryngeal vestibule or trachea [11]. No any outward signs of swallowing difficulty such as coughing during aspiration are called silent aspiration (similarly, silent penetration exists). Silent aspiration may be a result of pharyngeal musculature weakness, reduced laryngopharyngeal sensation, or impaired ability to produce a reflexive cough. Silent aspiration is often omitted even by medical professionals; many studies indicate that silent aspiration is associated with increased morbidity and mortality [12]. That is why dysphagia specialists emphasize the importance of dysphagia screening.

The words “laryngeal penetration” and “tracheal aspiration” have been used to show the difference between nasal regurgitation/penetration/aspiration during swallow.

However, recent evidence that the head of the bolus moves faster than the wave of pharyngeal contraction suggests that, at least in some situations, the kinetic energy imparted to the bolus as it is expelled from the mouth into the pharynx may be sufficient to carry it through the pharynx. The function of sequential contraction of the pharyngeal constrictor muscles may then be to facilitate subsequent pharyngeal clearance [13].

The styloglossus retracts and elevates the tongue in a posterior and superior fashion. Following mastication, these movements promote the passage of the food bolus towards the oropharynx. The hyoglossus and styloglossus are used (retract) during swallowing to push the bolus. Several exercises such as the supersupraglottic swallow, effortful swallow, Mendelsohn maneuver, and tongue-hold maneuver may improve tongue base retraction function [8, 14].

The deglutition reflex is initiated when the bolus passes through the junction of the oral cavity and pharynx and generates local afferent somatosensory inputs. Ice stimulation over the pharynx mucosa is a commonly-used method to facilitate the deglutition reflex. However, the deep somatosensory receptor should also be stimulated, that is, the tongue proprioceptor in the junction of the oral cavity and pharynx.

Some fibers of the palatoglossus spread over the dorsum of the tongue, others pass deeply into the substance of the tongue to intermingle with fibers of the intrinsic transverse muscle, thereby forming a muscular ring structure between the oral cavity and pharynx. We found that needle insertion into the tongue towards the junction of the oral cavity and pharynx can evoke the deglutition reflex. This finding indicates the important role of the tongue proprioceptor in this region in initiating the deglutition reflex.

Screening

Dysphagia can often be unnoticed/unreported because patients and clinicians are unfamiliar with symptoms and signs of dysphagia other than coughing during or after meal. Feeling difficulty when swallowing something or choking during a meal are easily identified symptoms of dysphagia. However, symptoms and signs of dysphagia may be slowing eating, weight loss, having bubbling sounds in the throat (feeling like phlegm) during or after a meal, feeling residue food left in the throat, feeling food retained in the esophagus, having difficulty falling asleep because of coughing, or getting hoarse [15, 16]. When swallowed liquid/solid food enters the airway, no coughing or other obvious airway reaction (i.e., silent aspiration or penetration) is not an uncommon situation. Silent aspiration may have a prevalence up to 89% in patients presenting aspiration [17] and is associated with low ADL scores and high mortality in older inpatients with aspiration pneumonia [18]. Thus, it is crucial to identify the risks of dysphagia.

Both the Seirei questionnaire (also known as the Ohkuma Questionnaire) for dysphagia screening and the Eating Assessment Tool (EAT-10) can be used to screen people with dysphagia. The Seirei (Ohkuma) questionnaire was originally developed for dysphagia screening in patients with the neurovascular disease. The reliability of the questionnaire has also been confirmed among community-dwelling older adults [19]. Each of the 15 items on the scale is arranged in three levels (Severe, Moderate/Mild, No). Selecting a severe level for any of the 15 questions indicates the risk of dysphagia [16].

The EAT-10 was originally developed as a dysphagia outcome instrument, which could be rapidly administered and easily scored to assess symptom severity, quality of life, and treatment efficacy. It has been demonstrated for the ability to predict aspiration [20, 21]. The scale is a self-report instrument. Each of the 10 items on the scale is arranged in 5 numerical levels (0 = No problem, 4= Severe problem). An EAT-10 score of 3 or higher is abnormal [15].

Compared to the EAT-10, the Seirei/Ohkuma Questionnaire consists of more items/symptoms related to dysphagia, e.g., a history of pneumonia, having bubbling sounds in the throat (feeling like phlegm) during or after a meal or at other times, having the feeling that food was retained or got stuck in the esophagus, having difficulty falling asleep or waking up because of coughing, getting hoarse, and food or sour liquid going back into the throat from the stomach. These symptoms may be signs of dysphagia and the sensitivity of screening can be reduced if the symptoms are omitted. Thus, for screening dysphagia in the community, the Seirei/Ohkuma Questionnaire can be considered.

For hospitalized patients, the most useful factors for the presence of a high risk of aspiration were considered to be: any disturbance of consciousness level, wet voice, weak voluntary cough, cough on drinking small volumes of water, and a timed water swallowing test[22-26]. These can be used as a very brief tool for dysphagia screening [27].

Note that weak/no voluntary cough is judged only when a patient actively initiates a cough following an order. Some patients exhibit intense coughing but cannot follow instruction to cough, which should be judged as no voluntary cough.

Compared to water, citric acid causes a stronger sensory stimulation to the airway wall. Thus, swallowing the citric acid solution is more sensitive to detect silent aspiration or penetration. That is, a patient without a cough reflex during/after drinking water (silent aspiration or penetration) may cough when drinking 2% w/v citric acid solution [17]. Hence, the citric acid solution swallowing test may replace a water swallowing test for screening dysphagia, especially when there is a shortage of medical professionals specialized in dysphagia care and minor responses of aspiration or penetration are hard to recognize.

A sequential water swallowing test

Water swallowing tests are common methods for evaluating swallowing function. After swallowing different volumes of water such as 3 ml (Modified water swallow test), 30 ml (Kubota Water Swallowing Test), or 90 ml (3-Oz water swallow test), the responses of the subject can be classified into three groups on the basis of the time course of swallowing though some symptoms may occur in all stages (**Table 1**). For example, coughing may be evoked when swallowed materials enter the airway during or after swallowing, whereas in the initiation stage premature loss of materials to be swallowed can enter the airway to cause coughing.

Table 1. Abnormal signs of dysphagia for water swallow tests

Initiation stage	During swallowing	Post swallowing
coughing	coughing	coughing
delayed initiating of swallowing	faster breathing	wet voice
unable to initiate swallowing	increased heart rate	throat clearing
food leaking out from oral cavity	drinking from a cup with interruption (for 30 ml or 90 ml)	faster breathing
		increased heart rate

We recommend a 1-3-5-10-30-90 ml sequence for performing a water swallowing test (**Figure 1**). For a small or medium volume ($\leq$ 10 ml), two to three repetitions are needed. The 30 ml or 90 ml volumes are tested once. For each tested volume, any symptom listed in **Table 1** indicates the possibility of dysphagia, especially an abnormal pharyngeal phase of swallowing. The 1-3-5-10-30-90 ml sequence includes the 3 ml (Modified water swallow test), 30 ml (Kubota Water Swallowing Test), and 90 ml (**3-Oz water swallow test**) water swallow tests. Here, Table 1 provides a consistent standard. The algorithm to perform the water swallow test is shown as follows (**Figure 1**):

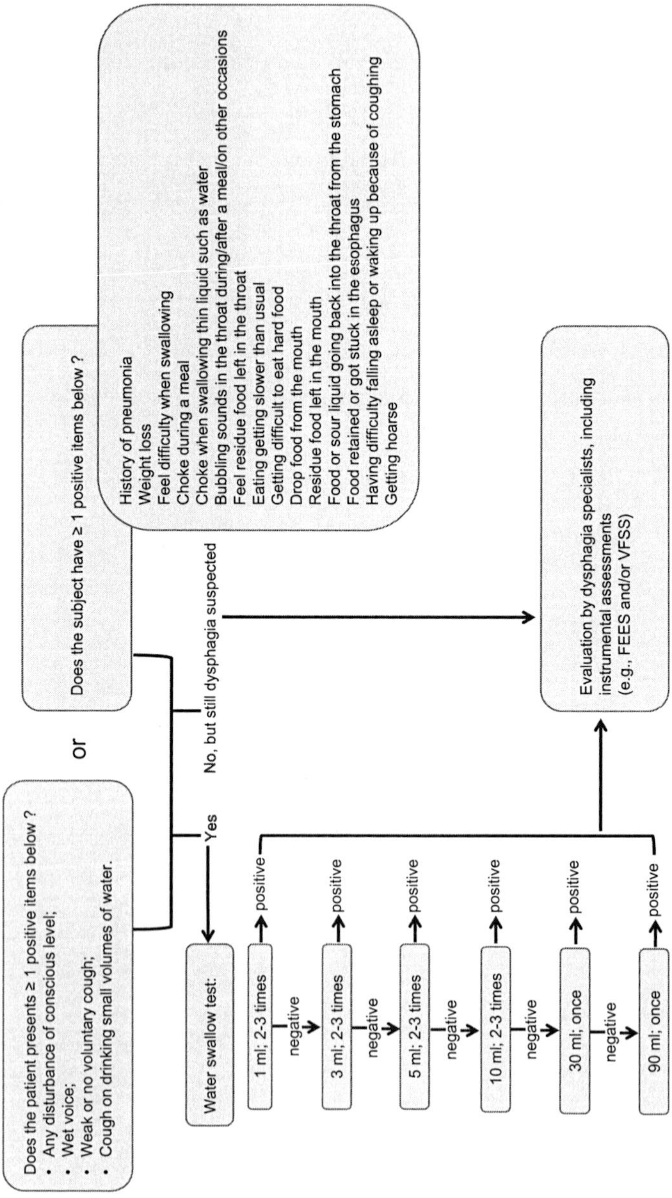

Figure 1 A sequential water swallowing test

The sequential water swallowing test has several merits. First, a gradual increase from a small amount takes into account safety issues. A higher volume is tested only when no positive response is observed.

Additionally, for all tested volumes, Table 1 provides a consistent standard, which consists of criteria in the 3 ml (Modified water swallow test), 30 ml (Kubota Water Swallowing Test), and 90 ml (3-Oz water swallow test) water swallow tests. The listed positive responses during a given volume indicate the possibility of dysphagia and thus the subject needs to be evaluated by specialists.

Semi-solid and solid food need to be tested by dysphagia specialists in that these materials may cause asphyxia.

Using pulse oximeter

Simultaneous usage of a pulse oximeter during a water swallow test can detect changes in the oxygen desaturation and heart rate. A decrease in SpO2 exceeding 2% or 3% is considered desaturation caused by aspiration, which still lacks consistent evidence. Note that aspiration does not necessarily lead to a decrease in blood oxygen level, especially when obvious airway responses (e.g., coughing) are lacking. On the contrary, faster breathing after penetration/aspiration may slightly increase the blood oxygen level. Thus, we recommend observing the baseline blood oxygen level and heart rate for one minute before a water swallow test, and then note whether there are post-swallowing changes (either an increase or decrease) beyond the magnitude during the baseline period [28, 29].

This procedure may provide useful information for patients with language dysfunction, cognitive impairment, or weak/no voluntary cough.

Wet voice

A wet voice may indicate dysphagia but not aspiration.

A wet voice after swallowing is a common sign used to judge whether a subject has a risk of dysphagia. A wet voice means a liquid sounding, that is, a sounding being produced through moisture. Presumably, poor pharyngeal clearance lead to accumulated saliva or swallowed fluid in the pyriform sinuses or on the vocal cords, which are the sources of the moisture and result in a wet quality of the voice [29].

The value of a wet voice is controversial. For example, a wet voice when phonating “ah” after swallowing (counting from 1 to 5) was not found to be associated with penetration or aspiration after ingesting liquid or pudding [29], but a wet voice when phonating [ε] after swallowing indicates penetration or aspiration in patients with Parkinson's disease in case of a positive test [30].

To address whether a wet voice is a useful sign and how to effectively examine a wet voice, the possible mechanisms of a wet voice should be analyzed. A wet voice may be produced under two conditions. One possibility is fluid accumulation (swallowed liquid, or saliva) on the vocal cords after swallowing, that is, the outside fluid enters the larynx (because of penetration or aspiration) and moistens the vocal cords. The other condition is secretions discharged from the airway after penetration/aspiration, which causes a liquid sounding. Under such conditions, tracheal secretions or secretions from laryngeal glands. Age-related changes in the distribution of laryngeal glands in the human adult larynx are generated due to stimulation by materials entering the airway [31]. That is, the liquid is the secretion by the larynx/trachea rather than swallowed materials. Numerous mucous glands exist on the laryngeal mucosa, distributed over the epiglottis and margins of the aryepiglottic folds. During phonation, some large glands in the saccules of the larynx secrete periodically over the vocal cords. These glands are the sources of secretion [9].

When the "thin liquid," "nectar," or "honey" cover the vocal folds during phonation, the higher frequency harmonics are suppressed whereas intermittent additional frequencies in the low and high end of the acoustic spectrum are generated (but the three fluid conditions may not be easily differentiated). These are the acoustic mechanisms of the wet voice [32]. After swallowing, both foreign materials entering the larynx and secretions from laryngeal glands or the trachea can be sources of the liquid moistening the vocal cords. Using laryngeal endoscopy, mildly thick and severely thick mucus aggregation may be observed on the vocal folds [33].

When performing FEES, a wet voice or even blister sounds can be found when the fluid is accumulated over the vocal cords after swallowing. That is a direct view of why the voice is "wet". Thus, detecting a wet voice needs several conditions: 1) if the voice is not wet before swallowing, the pre-swallow voice and post-swallow voice can be compared to examine whether the voice becomes "wet". 2) The swallowed material should be a thin liquid (e.g., water) since a thin liquid is more likely to enter the larynx and is accumulated on the vocal cords to let the voice be "wet" in comparison with solid food or semi-solid food. Note that penetration may occur in healthy people but hardly reach the vocal cords [11]. A voice with sufficient vocal-cords vibration should be used to examine wet voice. That is, phonating a vowel sound. Different vowels such as /i:/, /ɑ:/, and /e/ have been used in previous studies where which one is better is not determined. 4) phonating a voice should last a long duration if possible, but a short period may be enough to detect a wet voice.

Thus, the recommended steps to check a wet voice are:

1) Ask the patient to say /i:/ 2 times before swallowing;
2) Ask the patient to swallow a given amount of water,
3) Immediately after swallowing, ask the patient to say /i:/ 2 times, any changes in the tone/quality of the voice are abnormal. Note a patient may not be able to phonate a long vowel, and thus the changes during a brief pronunciation of a vowel should be noticed.

FEES (Flexible Endoscopic Evaluation of Swallowing)

Both FEES and VFSS are gold standards to evaluate dysphagia. Compared to VFSS, FESS can directly view the 3D dynamics of the laryngeal inlet during swallowing, which is a unique benefit. During swallow, the laryngeal inlet and the vocal cords are closed to prevent food from entering the airway. These laryngeal closures can be viewed with FEES. The vocal cords abduction/adduction can be seen in a posterior-anterior position during VFSS, whereas movements of the laryngeal inlet (mainly aryepiglottic fold) are hardly visible during VFSS. In addition, FEES has no ionizing radiation and can be performed with a portable instrument and thus can be implemented in various environments including inpatient wards and nursing homes.

The disadvantages of FEES include invisibility of the pharyngeal phase, insufficient exposure of airways under the vocal cords, and occlusion of the lens field of view by secretions during examination. VFSS can view the oral cavity, pharynx, larynx, and the upper part of the esophagus in one field of view but FEES cannot.

Inserting a flexible laryngoscope using a 3-ortho principle

For many beginners, FEES insertion may encounter difficulties. When the patient is in a seated position, the core points of inserting the flexible laryngoscope are keeping the ortho-positions of the operator, patient, and tube. These points can be called a "3 ortho" principle for insertion. The ortho-position of the operator/patient indicates that the head needs to face straight ahead (without turning around). The insertion (anterior) part of the tube should also be kept in an ortho-position, that is, the tube should be positioned/moved along the extension line of the lower nasal meatus (i.e., parallel to the middle sagittal plane and along the floor of the lower nasal meatus) when the insertion is started.

For beginners, it is easier to insert the tube through the lower nasal meatus under most conditions. Holding the tube with a hand at the position approximately 15-20 cm from the front end. Advance the tube along the floor of the lower nasal meatus (towards the darkest direction). Avoid touching the tissues (obstacles) by the tip of the tube. Slightly adjusting the direction of the tube front end if any tissues (obstacles) are seen directly in front of the tube front end on the monitor; adjusting the direction can be achieved through 1) moving the hand holding the tube, 2) bending the tube front end, and/or 3) rotating the tube. Small amplitudes of adjusting are often enough. A very common mistake is to bend the front end of the tube too much when advancing the tube. Except for the nasopharynx, in other positions, the tube does not need to be bent at a large angle.

For a successful insertion, it is essential to understand the spatial relations among the lower nasal meatus, the tube, the operator, and the patient. The 3-ortho principle for insertion is a simple way to arrange these spatial relations.

The front end of the fiberoptic endoscope should be lubricated (e.g., with a nonanaesthetic or anesthetic gel) before passing trans-nasally, especially for a dry nasal cavity. Spraying or spreading 1% tetracaine/lidocaine solution in the nasal cavity and pharynx is not recommended.

In our patients, applying anesthetic gel on the tube appears to have no effects on the movement of the soft palate, pharynx, and larynx, possibly due to 1) the amount of the applied anesthetic gel is small, and 2) during FEES, only part of the applied gel over the tube is separated from the tube and then contact pharyngeal/laryngeal tissues.

Using starch as the dye in FEES

Dyed food (liquid, semi-solid, and solid) is often used in FEES to improve the visibility of swallowed material. Blue, green, or white-colored or –dyed food presents good contrast to pharyngeal/laryngeal tissues, whereas a color similar to the mucous membrane of the pharynx/larynx (e.g., pink or red) cannot be used to dye food. FEES presents both high intra- and interrater reliability in detecting bolus retention, laryngeal penetration, and tracheal aspiration using either yellow-colored pudding and white-colored milk or blue-dyed pudding/milk [34].

When using food coloring (blue dye or green dye) or methylene blue during FEES, absorption of the swallowed dye may lead to side effects in some patients. Colored food, e.g., white milk or yellow pudding can present good contrast in FEES. Some people may be allergic to milk. Barium liquid presents white color and is thus used in some institutes, but it may lead to constipation. Additionally, barium may be deposited in the trachea/lung after laryngeal aspiration, which is hardly cleared.

Thus, we recommend using edible starch as the dye in FEES. Starch can be easily acquired. The starch solution is white-colored, non-allergic to most people, and easier to be discharged from the trachea in comparison with barium. The starch solution is a type of thin liquid and can be thickened to prepare nectar-thick and spoon-thick liquids, and white-colored pudding.

Starch is a polysaccharide substance and is insoluble in cold water. Starch dissolved in hot water becomes a viscous translucent colloidal solution, which is thicker than a cold starch solution. Therefore, for preparing thin liquids with a viscosity close to that of water, the starch solution should be made at room temperature or lower (e.g., below 24 degrees Celsius). The solubility of different types of starch varies. Enough starch should be added to the water to prepare a milky white solution.

Thickener can be used to prepare nectar-like and spoon-thick liquids. For pudding and solid food, use those that contrast sharply with the color of the mucous membranes, e.g., white or yellow.

Infection control of FEES

Over the course of FEES, body fluids and contaminants contaminate the external surface and internal channels of the flexible endoscope, which may lead to endoscopic transmission of infection if insufficient cleaning and disinfection (or sterilization) are performed. *Cleaning* physically removes organic and other materials by using a multi-enzyme solution or other detergent solutions but does not kill them. *Disinfection* destroys most microorganisms usually by using liquid chemical disinfectants (e.g., ≥2% glutaral solution≥10min); there are 3 levels of disinfection (high, intermediate, and low), and high-level disinfection eradicates vegetative microorganisms, mycobacteria, fungi, nonlipid (nonenveloped) and lipid viruses through bacterial spores may not be killed. *Sterilization* can eliminate all microbes including bacterial spores with heat, ethylene oxide gas, or ≥2% glutaral solution ≥10 h [35].

A flexible endoscope contacts intact mucous membrane and does not penetrate tissues during FEES procedures. It should receive high-level disinfection or sterilization after each use [35, 36].

To ensure the flexible endoscope is safe for patient use, reprocessing this equipment should consistently follow a number of essential steps (below is an example of steps for a flexible endoscope without an internal channel) [35-37]:

1) Pre-cleaning: perform pre-cleaning *immediately* after completing the FEES procedure, e.g., wipe the operating part and the tube with gauze pads containing multi-enzyme solution. A multi-enzyme cleaner can quickly decompose various organic secretions and thus help to remove microorganisms from the surface of the endoscope. This is critical for preventing the formation of biofilm, a matrix of extracellular polymeric substances covering microbial cells that adhere to each other on the tube surface.
2) Leak testing: this step should be performed after pre-cleaning and prior to manual cleaning. In this step, damage of the external surfaces and internal channels of the endoscope can be detected. These problems may lead to damage of the endoscope during the next steps.
3) Manual cleaning: soak the endoscope in multi-enzyme solution for 4 min, and then brush and flush the tube to eliminate organic material by using a multi-enzyme solution.
4) Rinsing: flush the endoscope with flowing water to completely evacuate liquid chemical germicides.
5) Visual inspection: using lighted magnification visually inspect the endoscope and its accessories to assure that the instrument is clean.
6) Disinfection or sterilization: soak the endoscope with ≥2% pH 7.5-8.5 glutaral solution ≥ 10min for disinfection, ≥ 45 min for destroying Hepatitis B virus and mycobacterium, or ≥ 10 h for sterilization. Assure that the endoscope has been dried before soaking. Otherwise, the concentration of the glutaral solution will be reduced.
7) Rinsing and drying: flush the endoscope with flowing sterilized water and then with 70% alcohol solution. The 70% alcohol flush can promote drying of the endoscope and inhibit the growth of organisms.

Drying the endoscope after rinsing.

A promising technique: oropharyngeal electrical-vibration stimulation

We develop an oropharyngeal electrical-vibration stimulation technique that can improve swallowing function better than electrical stimulation or vibration stimulation alone. The method stimulates the tongue, buccinator, and other muscles around the mouth and cheeks (those moving cheeks, lips and oral fissure, the oral vestibule, and the jaws), soft palate, and lateral and posterior walls of the pharynx with concurrent vibration stimulation and low-frequency pulse electrical current (0-1000Hz). For vibration, low frequencies and higher levels (e.g., 0-5000 Hz) may be applied. When using electrical current at the same magnitude, that plus concurrent vibration stimulation evokes a stronger sensation.

The electrical stimulation is performed by using a spoon-shaped electrode and a surface electrode. The surface electrode is attached to the skin between the mandibular and thyroid cartilage (a needle electrode may be better; inserting the needle towards the root of the tongue until a swallowing movement is evoked and then fixing the needle with tape). The spoon-shaped electrode enters the oral cavity and then contacts a place on the inner surface of the oropharyngeal cavity. Vibration stimulation is achieved by using a vibrator attached to the handle of the spoon-shaped electrode. The frequency and intensity of vibration and electrical current can be modulated separately.

Place the spoon-shaped electrode at the center of the tongue. Then, initiate electrical stimulation and gradually increase the intensity until the patient has weak electrical pulse sensations. Afterwards, initiate vibration stimulation and gradually increase the intensity to a tolerated level. Slowly move the spoon-shaped electrode over the tongue, soft palate, muscles moving the lips and cheek, and lateral and posterior walls of the pharynx. Depending on the patient's tolerance, the intensity of the stimulation can be increased gradually.

During stimulation, spontaneous swallowing may be observed. After stimulation for tens of seconds, remove the spoon-shaped electrode out of the mouth, ask the patient to try to perform dry swallow one or more times, and then restart stimulation. A session usually lasts 10-20 min. One or two sessions may be performed per day.

The oropharyngeal electrical-vibration stimulation can activate paralyzed muscles of the oropharyngeal cavity, including those responsible for transporting the bolus and participating in the swallow reflex occurring in the pharyngeal phase of the swallow. Especially, the method can activate suprahyoid muscles and facilitate anterior-forward movement of the hyoid-larynx complex.

A number of muscles are involved in swallowing movement. This stimulation technique activates many of these muscles; it can further focus on strengthening key factors (e.g., timely and strong tongue base retraction for the pharyngeal phase). For a complex process such as swallowing, improvement of a key neuro-biomechanical component may drive functional normalization of other components.

This non-invasive stimulation technique can improve swallowing function via enhancing somatosensory inputs, facilitating muscle contraction, and modulating brain function. Additionally, stimulating tongue muscles has been shown to be able to improve cognitive function in brain injury patients [38]. Therefore, the oropharyngeal electrical-vibration stimulation may have a broad spectrum of treatment effects on a number of neurological diseases.

Balloon-catheter dilation for treating UES dysfunction

When swallowing a large bolus, passive opening of the UES (relying on the elasticity of the UES) and the pressure of the bolus occurs earlier than force generation by contractions of suprahyoid muscles [39], suggesting that stretching (e.g., dilating the UES with an inflated balloon) may correct decreased elasticity as an intervention to address UES narrowing. The balloon dilation is a minimally invasive procedure and can be performed by using a dual-lumen Foley catheter with a balloon.

The dilation procedure is as follows (remove the nasogastric feeding tube if existing):

1) Inject 10mL water into the balloon to check whether the balloon is intact.

2) Lubricated the catheter with a nonanaesthetic or anesthetic gel.

3) Insert the catheter into the esophagus through the nose or mouth. The mouth is preferred if the patient is tolerated. The nasal cavity (if via the nose) or throat (if via the mouth) may be numbed by spraying anesthetic drugs, e.g., 1% tetracaine/lidocaine.

4) After the catheter passes through the UES (generally, the insertion length is no less than 30 cm), soak the external end of the catheter in the water to check whether air bubbles appear. At the same time, observe whether the patient suffers cyanosis and/or dyspnea.

5) Inject 6-9 ml of water into the balloon by using a syringe. When the patient receives this dilation procedure for the first time, the volume of injected water should be increased slowly to determine the maximum volume that the patient can tolerate. Depending on the extent of UES narrowing, this maximum volume varies from person to person and may be as low as 2 mL.

6) Ask the patient to indicate the position of the inflated balloon with a finger.

7) An operator gently pulled up the inflated balloon until it is blocked by the narrowed segment while the other operator continuously holds the syringe (otherwise, the water will flow back to the syringe from the balloon due to pressure). Ask the patient to indicate the current position of the inflated balloon with a finger to check whether it reaches the level of the UES (slightly below the thyroid bone).

8) Gradually increase the pulling force if the patient can tolerate it. Any pain should be avoided.

9) Hold the tensioned catheter for up to 2 min, or pull up the catheter and then relax repeatedly until the balloon is passed through the cricopharyngeal muscle. If the procedure is performed via the nose, the injected water should be drawn out of the balloon as soon as the balloon is passed through the cricopharyngeal muscle. Otherwise, the balloon may be

blocked by the nasal cavity. Note that there may not be a sensation of resistance reduction when the balloon is passed the UES. Thus, always ask the patient to indicate the position of the inflated balloon during pulling, especially when the balloon reaches the level of the cricopharyngeal muscle. Note that during the procedure, some patients cannot clearly differentiate whether the inflated balloon is blocked by the UES or by the nasal cavity.

10) Repeat steps 2-9, up to 6 times in a treatment session if the patient can tolerate it. Gradually increase the volume of the balloon dilation (usually, 0.5-1 mL each time). After dilation, nebulized inhalation (e.g., with dexamethasone or budesonide) may be given to prevent mucosal edema and reduce mucus secretion.

11) Avoid any pain in the pharynx, UES, and esophagus when dilating and pulling up the balloon. Before performing the procedure, tell the patient to present a signal, e.g., hand waving, as soon as feeling throat or chest pain during the dilation and pulling-up.

12) The procedure may be performed one session per day or per every other day based on the patient's tolerance.

After the catheter is inserted into the esophagus through the nose or mouth, the balloon is inflated with normal saline at a suitable volume (depending on the extent of UES narrowing). Then, the inflated catheter is gently pulled up until it is blocked by the narrowed segment [40-44].

The position where the balloon is blocked is the caudal end of UES dysfunction [44, 45], which can be visualized via ultrasonography.

References

[1] Takizawa C, Gemmell E, Kenworthy J, Speyer R. A Systematic Review of the Prevalence of Oropharyngeal Dysphagia in Stroke, Parkinson's Disease, Alzheimer's Disease, Head Injury, and Pneumonia. Dysphagia. 2016; 31: 434-41 – 10.1007/s00455-016-9695-9 [doi].

[2] Espinosa-Val MC, Martín-Martínez A, Graupera M, et al. Prevalence, Risk Factors, and Complications of Oropharyngeal Dysphagia in Older Patients with Dementia. Nutrients. 2020; 12.

[3] Aldridge KJ, Taylor NF. Dysphagia is a common and serious problem for adults with mental illness: a systematic review. Dysphagia. 2012; 27: 124-37.

[4] Madhavan A, LaGorio LA, Crary MA, Dahl WJ, Carnaby GD. Prevalence of and Risk Factors for Dysphagia in the Community Dwelling Elderly: A Systematic Review. J Nutr Health Aging. 2016; 20: 806-815.

[5] Jadcherla S. Dysphagia in the high-risk infant: potential factors and mechanisms. Am J Clin Nutr. 2016; 103: 622S-8S.

[6] Almirall J, Rofes L, Serra-Prat M, et al. Oropharyngeal dysphagia is a risk factor for community-acquired pneumonia in the elderly. Eur Respir J. 2013; 41: 923-8.

[7] Kohno A, Kohno M, Ohkoshi S. Swallowing and aspiration during sleep in patients with obstructive sleep apnea versus control individuals. Sleep. 2022; 45.

[8] Andaloro C, Sharma P, La Mantia I. Anatomy, Head and Neck, Larynx Arytenoid Cartilage. 2022. Treasure Island (FL). StatPearls

Publishing.

[9] Standring S. Gray's Anatomy. 2004. 39. UK. Churchill Livingstone. 641-642.

[10] Rosenbek JC, Robbins JA, Roecker EB, Coyle JL, Wood JL. A penetration-aspiration scale. Dysphagia. 1996; 11: 93-8.

[11] Robbins J, Coyle J, Rosenbek J, Roecker E, Wood J. Differentiation of normal and abnormal airway protection during swallowing using the penetration-aspiration scale. Dysphagia. 1999; 14: 228-32.

[12] Ramsey D, Smithard D, Kalra L. Silent aspiration: what do we know. Dysphagia. 2005; 20: 218-25.

[13] Standring S. Gray's Anatomy. 2004. 39. UK. Churchill Livingstone. 336-586.

[14] Gassert RB, Pearson WG Jr. Evaluating muscles underlying tongue base retraction in deglutition using muscular functional magnetic resonance imaging (mfMRI). Magn Reson Imaging. 2016; 34: 204-8.

[15] Lechien JR, Cavelier G, Thill MP, et al. Validity and reliability of the French version of Eating Assessment Tool (EAT-10). Eur Arch Otorhinolaryngol. 2019; 276: 1727-1736.

[16] Ohkuma R, Fujishima I, Kojima C, Hojo K, Takehara I, Motohashi Y. Development of a questionnaire to screen dysphagia. Jpn J Dysphagia Rehabil. 2002; 6: 3-8.

[17] Velayutham P, Irace AL, Kawai K, et al. Silent aspiration: Who is at risk. Laryngoscope. 2018; 128: 1952-1957.

[18] Nakashima T, Maeda K, Tahira K, et al. Silent aspiration predicts mortality in older adults with aspiration pneumonia admitted to

acute hospitals. Geriatr Gerontol Int. 2018; 18: 828-832.

[19] Kawashima K, Motohashi Y, Fujishima I. Prevalence of dysphagia among community-dwelling elderly individuals as estimated using a questionnaire for dysphagia screening. Dysphagia. 2004; 19: 266-71.

[20] Rofes L, Arreola V, Mukherjee R, Clavé P. Sensitivity and specificity of the Eating Assessment Tool and the Volume-Viscosity Swallow Test for clinical evaluation of oropharyngeal dysphagia. Neurogastroenterol Motil. 2014; 26: 1256-65.

[21] Cheney DM, Siddiqui MT, Litts JK, Kuhn MA, Belafsky PC. The Ability of the 10-Item Eating Assessment Tool (EAT-10) to Predict Aspiration Risk in Persons With Dysphagia. Ann Otol Rhinol Laryngol. 2015; 124: 351-4.

[22] Mélotte E, Maudoux A, Delhalle S, et al. Swallowing in individuals with disorders of consciousness: A cohort study. Ann Phys Rehabil Med. 2021; 64: 101403.

[23] Smithard DG, O'Neill PA, Park C, et al. Can bedside assessment reliably exclude aspiration following acute stroke. Age Ageing. 1998; 27: 99-106.

[24] Kidd D, Lawson J, Nesbitt R, MacMahon J. Aspiration in acute stroke: a clinical study with videofluoroscopy. Q J Med. 1993; 86: 825-9.

[25] Gottlieb D, Kipnis M, Sister E, Vardi Y, Brill S. Validation of the 50 ml3 drinking test for evaluation of post-stroke dysphagia. Disabil Rehabil. 1996; 18: 529-32.

[26] Hinds NP, Wiles CM. Assessment of swallowing and referral to speech and language therapists in acute stroke. QJM. 1998; 91:

829-35.

[27] O'Neill PA. Swallowing and prevention of complications. Br Med Bull. 2000；56: 457-65.

[28] Britton D, Roeske A, Ennis SK, Benditt JO, Quinn C, Graville D. Utility of Pulse Oximetry to Detect Aspiration: An Evidence-Based Systematic Review. Dysphagia. 2018；33: 282-292.

[29] Wang TG, Chang YC, Chen SY, Hsiao TY. Pulse oximetry does not reliably detect aspiration on videofluoroscopic swallowing study. Arch Phys Med Rehabil. 2005；86: 730-4.

[30] Sampaio M, Argolo N, Melo A, Nóbrega AC. Wet voice as a sign of penetration/aspiration in Parkinson's disease: does testing material matter. Dysphagia. 2014；29: 610-5.

[31] Tomita H, Nakashima T, Maeda A, Umeno H, Sato K. Age related changes in the distribution of laryngeal glands in the human adult larynx. Auris Nasus Larynx. 2006；33: 289-94.

[32] Murugappan S, Boyce S, Khosla S, Kelchner L, Gutmark E. Acoustic characteristics of phonation in "wet voice" conditions. J Acoust Soc Am. 2010；127: 2578-89.

[33] Bonilha HS, White L, Kuckhahn K, Gerlach TT, Deliyski DD. Vocal fold mucus aggregation in persons with voice disorders. J Commun Disord. 2012；45: 304-11.

[34] Leder SB, Acton LM, Lisitano HL, Murray JT. Fiberoptic endoscopic evaluation of swallowing (FEES) with and without blue-dyed food. Dysphagia. 2005；20: 157-62.

[35] ASGE Quality Assurance in Endoscopy Committee, Calderwood AH, Day LW, et al. ASGE guideline for infection control during GI endoscopy. Gastrointest Endosc. 2018；87: 1167-1179.

[36] China ShaFPCotpRo. Regulation for cleaning and disinfeciton technique of flexible endoscope. WS 507-2016,2017. 13.

[37] Committee HICPA. Essential Elements of a Reprocessing Program for Flexible Endoscopes – The Recommendations of the Healthcare Infection Control Practices Advisory Committee (HICPAC) ,2016.

[38] Danilov Y, Paltin D. Translingual Neurostimulation (TLNS): Perspective on a Novel Approach to Neurorehabilitation after Brain Injury. New York, NY,2018.

[39] Cock C, Jones CA, Hammer MJ, Omari TI, McCulloch TM. Modulation of Upper Esophageal Sphincter (UES) Relaxation and Opening During Volume Swallowing. Dysphagia. 2017； 32: 216-224.

[40] Xie M, Zeng P, Wan G, et al. The Effect of Combined Guidance of Botulinum Toxin Injection with Ultrasound, Catheter Balloon, and Electromyography on Neurogenic Cricopharyngeal Dysfunction: A Prospective Study. Dysphagia. 2021； .

[41] Chen JM, Chen YJ, Ni J, Wang ZY. Ultrasound, electromyography, and balloon guidance for injecting botulinum toxin for cricopharyngeal achalasia: A case report. Medicine (Baltimore). 2021； 100: e24909.

[42] Luan S, Wu SL, Xiao LJ, et al. Comparison studies of ultrasound-guided botulinum toxin injection and balloon catheter dilatation in the treatment of neurogenic cricopharyngeal muscle dysfunction. NeuroRehabilitation. 2021； 49: 629-639.

[43] Zhu L, Chen J, Shao X, et al. Botulinum toxin A injection using ultrasound combined with balloon guidance for the treatment of cricopharyngeal dysphagia: analysis of 21 cases. Scand J

Gastroenterol. 2022；: 1-7.

[44] Wei P, Xu Y, Zhang Z, Zhang S, Lv Z. Treatment for upper esophageal sphincter dysfunction in a patient with poststroke dysphagia: A case report. Medicine (Baltimore). 2019; 98: e14988 - 10.1097/MD.0000000000014988 [doi].

[45] Huai J, Hou Y, Guan J, et al. Botulinum Toxin A Injection Using Esophageal Balloon Radiography Combined with CT Guidance for the Treatment of Cricopharyngeal Dysphagia. Dysphagia. 2020; 35: 630-635.